The OTA's Guide to Documentation

Writing SOAP Notes

Third Edition

The OTA's Guide to Documentation

Writing SOAP Notes

Third Edition

Marie J. Morreale, OTR/L, CHT
Adjunct Faculty
Rockland Community College
State University of New York
Suffern, New York

Sherry Borcherding, MA, OTR/L
Clinical Associate Professor, Retired
University of Missouri-Columbia
Columbia, Missouri

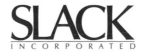

SLACK
INCORPORATED

Contents

Instructors: *The OTA's Guide to Documentation: Writing SOAP Notes, Third Edition Instructor's Manual* is also available from SLACK Incorporated. Don't miss this important companion to *The OTA's Guide to Documentation: Writing SOAP Notes, Third Edition*. To obtain the Instructor's Manual, please visit http://www.efacultylounge.com

Chapter 1

Documenting the Occupational Therapy Process

An occupational therapy assistant (OTA) has many roles and responsibilities, including the essential task of documenting occupational therapy services. In addition to writing in the health record, documentation also includes accurate recordkeeping for school, community, or nontraditional settings. Your professional documentation provides important information and feedback to the occupational therapist (OT) and treatment team regarding your clients. Initially, writing in the record might seem very intimidating to an OTA student or novice practitioner. When you first see an experienced OT or OTA make an entry in a health or education record, you might be tempted to think you will never be able to do it. Just the technical language alone can be daunting, and then there is the amazing attention to detail in the client observation, the insightful assessment, and the documentation that just seems to flow from the pen or computer keyboard without apparent effort. You may wonder whether you will be able to organize all of your client observations, predict what the next steps will be, and record interventions so quickly and professionally. You may also feel apprehensive because the process and terminology seem a little foreign to you. Rest assured that many occupational therapy practitioners felt the same way as you when they were students.

Professional documentation is a skill, and like any skill, it can be learned. Learning a skill, whether it is ice skating, playing the violin, or composing a progress note, requires three things of you: instruction, practice, and patience. This manual is designed to get you started with learning and practicing the process. Information is systematically provided on each part of the documentation process and the worksheets are designed to let you practice each step as you learn it. Use the manual as a workbook. Take time to integrate the information in each section, complete each exercise, and check it against the suggested answers in the Appendix. As you reflect and learn from your mistakes, you will develop confidence in your documentation abilities.

Overview

This manual presents a thorough and systematic approach to one form of documentation—the SOAP note. SOAP is an acronym for the four parts of an entry into the record. The letters stand for Subjective, Objective, Assessment, and Plan. You will learn the origins and meanings of those terms in Chapter 2, along with an explanation of an alternate format called a *narrative note*. The format this manual teaches for writing SOAP notes is one that is reimbursable by third-party payers, including Medicare, which has rigorous requirements. Not all funding sources require a SOAP note format and not all occupational therapy practitioners and facilities use SOAP notes. However, once you learn the basics for composing SOAP notes, you will then be able to adapt and apply those observation and documentation skills to other methods of recording client care (e.g., electronic formats, flow sheets, or

Morreale MJ, Borcherding S.
The OTA's Guide to Documentation:
Writing SOAP Notes, Third Edition (pp 1-10).
© 2013 SLACK Incorporated.

narrative notes) required by your medical facility, school, or other practice area. Also, if you learn to meet these strict standards, you are not likely to be denied reimbursement by any third-party payer. Current occupational therapy practice is in many ways determined by which services are reimbursable, and documentation of skilled client care is the method by which that service is communicated. Essentials of documentation, billing, and reimbursement are explained in Chapters 2 and 3. Those principles are also reflected in the many documentation examples presented throughout the manual. Each section of the SOAP note is also discussed thoroughly in separate chapters for the S, O, A, and P. In addition, this manual will help you to understand the purpose and standards of occupational therapy documentation for various practice settings and different stages of treatment. Other topics include electronic documentation, medical terminology, a review of grammar, an overview of the initial evaluation process delineating the roles of the OT and OTA, a method for writing goals, and guidelines for selecting appropriate interventions. The Appendix in this book provides suggested "answers" for the worksheets. However, as there are many "right" ways to answer, these must be viewed as suggestions rather than the only "correct" answers. In actual clinical practice, you will see varied documentation styles among occupational therapy practitioners. Each OT and OTA develops individualized writing skills and a personal repertoire of professional language while complying with accepted legal and facility standards.

This manual reflects the collaboration of the OT and OTA and incorporates standards of The American Occupational Therapy Association (AOTA) and the Accreditation Council for Occupational Therapy Education (ACOTE) for education, documentation, and clinical practice (ACOTE, 2012; AOTA 2008a, 2008b, 2009, 2010a, 2010c). The material presented in this book originally grew out of documentation courses taught to occupational therapy seniors at the University of Missouri-Columbia. The material was edited to be more appropriate for clinical practice of OTAs for the first edition of this book. The second and third editions incorporated new material that grew from documentation courses taught to OTA students at Rockland Community College, State University of New York. This edition reflects current guidelines for professional documentation and ethical clinical practice. The material has been field tested to be sure it is practical, understandable, and effective in helping you learn both documentation and clinical reasoning skills.

New in This Edition

This documentation manual has been revised to incorporate updated AOTA documents and standards for clinical practice. It reflects the scope of occupational therapy and emphasizes the basis of our services as described in the *Occupational Therapy Practice Framework: Domain and Process, 2nd Edition* (AOTA, 2008b). This manual also incorporates concepts and guidelines found in:

- *Guidelines for Documentation of Occupational Therapy* (AOTA, 2008a)
- *Guidelines for Supervision, Roles, and Responsibilities During the Delivery of Occupational Therapy Services* (AOTA, 2009)
- *Scope of Practice* (AOTA, 2010b)
- *Occupational Therapy Code of Ethics and Ethics Standards* (AOTA, 2010a)
- *Standards of Practice for Occupational Therapy* (AOTA, 2010c)
- *2011 Accreditation Council for Occupational Therapy Education (ACOTE) Standards* (ACOTE, 2012)
- *Occupational Therapy Services in the Promotion of Health and the Prevention of Disease and Disability* (AOTA, 2008c)

This *Third Edition* includes additional information on the mechanics of documentation, intervention planning, quality measures, electronic documentation, and narrative notes. A new billing and reimbursement chapter (with Medicare updates) and a new method of goal writing (COAST) are also included. Several tables have been added to help you develop observation skills and integrate professional language. The examples used in the text and worksheets are more diverse, with increased examples from mental health and pediatric practice settings. Chapters have been revised and reorganized to make the material current and easier to understand. New worksheets have been added or revised for optimal learning. For your convenience and additional practice, all worksheets in this *Third Edition* are now also available on a Web site. An Instructor's Manual has been created as an online resource to accompany this book and includes client treatment videos, grading rubrics, and additional learning activities for documentation.

Our Professional Language and Focus

International Classification of Functioning, Disability and Health

The *International Classification of Functioning, Disability and Health* (ICF) is a health and disability framework established by the World Health Organization (WHO) and endorsed by WHO members in 2001 (WHO, 2002, 2012b). ICF classifies, describes, and measures disability and health from the perspectives of not just physical health (pertaining to body structures and functions), but also a person's functional abilities (capacities) and actual performance levels for life tasks, while also considering the influence of social, personal, and environmental factors (WHO, 2002, 2012b). The standard, universal language of ICF pertains to individuals, institutions, and society and influences public policy. ICF posits that most individuals will experience some level of disability through declining health as a result of illness, injury, or the normal aging process (WHO, 2002, 2012b). Occupational therapy is a natural fit with the WHO viewpoint that health and disability are not solely based on a diagnosis but are impacted and intertwined with environmental factors, personal and social contexts, and actual abilities and limitations, all of which directly affect function, participation, and performance of life tasks (AOTA, 2008b; WHO, 2002, 2012b). It is useful to consider and incorporate terminology and concepts delineated in the ICF into your occupational therapy documentation.

Occupational Therapy Practice Framework

The *Occupational Therapy Practice Framework: Domain and Process, 2nd Edition* (AOTA, 2008b), also referred to as the *Framework-II*, is an important document that embodies the focus and heart of occupational therapy and is a useful resource for documenting professional terminology (Figure 1-1). The *Framework-II* describes the domain of occupational therapy as "supporting health and participation in life through engagement in occupation" (AOTA, 2008b, p. 626) and holistically delineates best practice for evaluation, intervention, and outcomes. This document presents a client-centered process that focuses on enabling individuals to perform desired life activities and meaningful occupations; the *Framework-II* groups these broad and varied life tasks into **areas of occupation** (AOTA, 2008b). The ability to engage in occupation is impacted by many interrelated factors: the client's **performance skills** (in the areas of motor and praxis, cognitive, sensory perceptual, communication and social, and emotional regulation); **performance patterns** (habits, routines, rituals and roles); **activity demands**; the influence of **context and environment**; and **client factors** (body structures and functions, spirituality, values and beliefs) (AOTA, 2008b). Your SOAP notes should reflect the professional occupational therapy language and concepts set forth by the *Framework-II*.

AREAS OF OCCUPATION	CLIENT FACTORS	PERFORMANCE SKILLS	PERFORMANCE PATTERNS	CONTEXT AND ENVIRONMENT	ACTIVITY DEMANDS
Activities of Daily Living (ADL)*	Values, Beliefs, and Spirituality	Sensory Perceptual Skills	Habits	Cultural	Objects Used and Their Properties
Instrumental Activities of Daily Living (IADL)	Body Functions	Motor and Praxis Skills	Routines	Personal	Space Demands
Rest and Sleep	Body Structures		Roles	Physical	Social Demands
Education		Emotional Regulation Skills	Rituals	Social	Sequencing and Timing
Work		Cognitive Skills		Temporal	Required Actions
Play		Communication and Social Skills		Virtual	Required Body Functions
Leisure					Required Body Structures
Social Participation					
*Also referred to as basic activities of daily living (BADL) or personal activities of daily living (PADL).					

Figure 1-1. Aspects of Occupational Therapy's Domain. (Reprinted with permission from American Occupational Therapy Association. (2008b). Occupational therapy practice framework: Domain and process (2nd ed.). *American Journal of Occupational Therapy, 62*(6), 625-683.)

By starting with an **occupational profile**, occupational therapy practitioners are able to determine whether any contextual or environmental features, activity demands, or individual client factors need to be addressed, depending on the occupational needs of the client (AOTA, 2008b). This allows appropriate goals and interventions to be determined for desired outcomes. The occupational profile is a client-centered approach to gathering information (occupational history, interests, experiences, habits, and patterns of daily living) as well as what the client values, needs, or hopes to gain from the present situation, allowing the client to set priorities for treatment (AOTA, 2008b). All of this initial data, plus any subsequent changes in the client's status, priorities, interventions, goals, and targeted outcomes, will be recorded in the different types of notes that occupational therapy practitioners write throughout the intervention process.

Influencing Contexts and Environments

The *Framework-II* also describes how clients engage in meaningful occupation in a variety of arenas called **contexts and environments** (AOTA, 2008b). In addition to internal and external contextual factors (e.g., age, gender, culture, socioeconomic status, developmental stages, temporal aspects), environments may be physical (e.g., home, school, climate, terrain), social (e.g., family, colleagues, church community); or virtual (e.g., the Internet) (AOTA, 2008b). If your client is being seen in an environment such as a hospital or clinic that is not usual for him or her, it is important to determine whether the skills you are teaching are transferable to his or her own environment. It is especially important to document how particular contexts and environments relate to the client's condition and may be barriers to occupational performance. For example, a client who has good functional mobility in the hospital may be completely stopped by three steps into a mobile home, an old fashioned bathtub on legs, or lack of an elevator at the job site. A client who lives in a rural area and can no longer drive may not have the option of public transportation for grocery shopping or getting to work. Due to peer pressure, a teenager may refuse to wear leg braces, wear hand splints, or use assistive devices. A recently retired executive may have difficulty adjusting to an abundance of leisure time. Your documentation should always include relevant contextual and environmental issues or problems along with any appropriate intervention or follow-up to address these situations.

Activity demands are interactive. They are most easily thought of in terms of task analysis. The demands of an activity include both what is needed to perform the activity and how that influences or relates to the client's stated goals.

Underlying Factors

The concepts of **client factors** and **performance skills** are sometimes confused when attempts are made to document a client's abilities and limitations. **Client factors** consist of **body structures and functions**, which refer to the client's anatomy and physiology, along with **spirituality, values, and beliefs**, which influence a client's meaning of life and motivation (AOTA, 2008b). For example, an amputation of a limb, a hysterectomy, or a dental extraction would be considered loss of a body structure. An adult with a degenerated hip joint or scoliosis or a child born with cleft palate, spina bifida, or club foot all have an impairment in a particular body structure. Body structures provide a physical framework to enable all of the body's systems to function, just like a water heater requires a metal container, pipes, nuts, and bolts before it can begin to work.

Some deficits in body structures can be "fixed" permanently or semi-permanently (total joint replacement, organ transplant, corrective surgery) or temporarily (dentures, prosthesis, wig). These "corrections" may sometimes necessitate a referral to occupational therapy. For example, intervention may include teaching compensatory dressing techniques following a total hip replacement, improving activity tolerance for a prosthesis, teaching energy conservation following a heart transplant, or improving mood or body image after a mastectomy.

The term *body functions* refers to making the body systems perform their duties, just like the water heater getting turned on and heating the water. Body functions include vital processes of basic life and movement functions such as breathing, righting reactions, reflexes, wound healing, digestion, and immunology (AOTA, 2008b). More overt body functions include areas such as strength, pain, the senses, and joint motion. Mental functions encompass cognitive and perceptual skills, and also include intrapersonal aspects such as personality, self-image, and emotions (AOTA, 2008b). If any of these client factors do not limit the client's ability to engage in desired occupational tasks, they do not necessarily need to be assessed or addressed in treatment. However, if a client has problems that do impact function such as poor memory, open wounds, dyspraxia, orthostatic hypotension, low vision, decreased strength, spasticity, low self-esteem, hallucinations, or anxiety, then these might be relevant client factors to document and target in your interventions.

Performance Skills

Occupational therapy practitioners use professional knowledge to assess the demands or requirements of activities and also to observe and analyze **performance skills**; these are client behaviors and actions grouped into five areas: **emotional regulation, motor and praxis, cognitive, sensory-perceptual,** and **communication and social** (AOTA, 2008b). As your client is performing activities, you will examine and document how those task skills are performed and consider what factors may impede function (AOTA, 2008b). For example, you can note the client's motor and praxis skills used to carry dishes to the table, reach to get clothes out of the dryer, push a shopping cart, manipulate knitting needles and yarn, bend to pick boxes up from the floor, grip pliers, or stand at a workstation for 10 minutes. Cognitive and sensory-perceptual skills are evident when you see a child, for example, put away the toys, play hopscotch, choose proper coins for the vending machine, attend to the math teacher, or organize a locker. You can note communication, social skills, and emotional regulation by observing the resident request a pain pill, express dissatisfaction about personal life decisions, ask for help with transfers, shake hands or make eye contact, speak in a low monotone voice, or share candy with others. You will be recording your professional observations and analysis of client behavior, actions, skills, and underlying client factors in your SOAP notes.

Engaging in Meaningful Occupation

Before we talk about documenting the occupational therapy process (Figure 1-2), we must differentiate occupational therapy from other health care disciplines. OTs and OTAs provide interventions for people who have problems engaging in an **area of occupation**. This is very important to note because this is what we will document. When documenting occupational therapy services, the focus on ability to engage in occupation is critical for demonstrating the necessity for occupational therapy and for preventing any question of duplication of services (Youngstrom, 2002). Occupational therapy practitioners in all service delivery settings have this common goal of facilitating occupational role performance (Youngstrom, 2002). It is also important to understand that each funding source has an interest in different outcomes or areas of occupation, meaning that payers have specific guidelines for what services they allow or consider necessary and will reimburse. This includes the specific type of occupational therapy interventions, frequency and duration of therapy, or any special equipment clients may need (e.g., hospital beds, splints, adaptive equipment, assistive technology, customized wheelchairs). Your documentation should reflect those payer interests and requirements as they pertain to the client's condition and needs, living environment/contexts, and realistic expected outcomes. For example, Worker's Compensation will be interested in a client's ability to return to work, Medicare may be concerned about a home care client's ability to perform ADLs safely at home, whereas a school district will be concerned about a child's ability to perform educationally related tasks as per the Individualized Education Program (IEP). The *Framework-II* describes the following eight areas of occupation (AOTA, 2008b):

Activities of Daily Living

Basic or personal activities of daily living (BADLs or PADLs) are necessary tasks for self-care and personal independence. These are tasks such as bathing, grooming, hygiene, dressing, eating, toileting, sexual activity, and functional mobility (AOTA, 2008b). It is important to consider not just the physical ability to care for self, but also other components, such as cognitive deficits or mental health conditions that might cause limitations in performance. For example, rather than being unable to perform grooming skills due to a physical factor, a client might fail to notice that his poor hygiene is problematic or he might be depressed and unmotivated to perform self-care. If your services are being reimbursed by Medicare, you will often find yourself writing goals for ADLs. For children, you will address ADLs as developmentally appropriate.

Instrumental Activities of Daily Living

Instrumental activities of daily living (IADLs) require more complex problem solving and social skills. IADLs include such tasks as money management, cleaning, laundry, child care, driving, shopping, and meal preparation (AOTA, 2008b). While these are necessary skills in adulthood, IADLs are also important developmental milestones for children and teenagers and can include caring for a pet, managing an allowance, babysitting, and using a microwave or stove. Occupational therapy practitioners who work with persons with brain injuries also consider executive functions that are an issue in frontal lobe damage. Executive functions involve planning, goal setting, and organizational tasks, which impact the ability to effectively perform IADLs. If your client population has cognitive impairment or mental health problems, you may find that your goals include multiple IADLs.

Work

Work includes successfully seeking and carrying out paid employment, as well as participating in volunteer experiences and planning for retirement (AOTA, 2008b). Work is a primary area of occupation for adults, forms a part of adult identity, and helps to structure one's day. If your services are being reimbursed by Workers' Compensation, you will find that the client's goals and interventions center around the return to work. Other work goals might include injury prevention such as ergonomics, safety education, and the elimination of hazards. If vocational rehabilitation is your funding source, you might find instead that your work goals involve helping prepare a client for work that is both meaningful and within the client's capabilities.

EVALUATION
Occupational profile—The initial step in the evaluation process that provides an understanding of the client's occupational history and experiences, patterns of daily living, interests, values, and needs. The client's problems and concerns about performing occupations and daily life activities are identified, and the client's priorities are determined.
Analysis of occupational performance—The step in the evaluation process during which the client's assets, problems, or potential problems are more specifically identified. Actual performance is often observed in context to identify what supports performance and what hinders performance. Performance skills, performance patterns, context or contexts, activity demands, and client factors are all considered, but only selected aspects may be specifically assessed. Targeted outcomes are identified.

INTERVENTION
Intervention plan—A plan that will guide actions taken and that is developed in collaboration with the client. It is based on selected theories, frames of reference, and evidence. Outcomes to be targeted are confirmed.
Intervention implementation—Ongoing actions taken to influence and support improved client performance. Interventions are directed at identified outcomes. Client's response is monitored and documented.
Intervention review—A review of the implementation plan and process as well as its progress toward targeted outcomes.

OUTCOMES (Supporting Health and Participation in Life Through Engagement in Occupation)
Outcomes—Determination of success in reaching desired targeted outcomes. Outcome assessment information is used to plan future actions with the client and to evaluate the service program (i.e., program evaluation).

Figure 1-2. Process of Service Delivery. (Reprinted with permission from American Occupational Therapy Association. (2008b). Occupational therapy practice framework: Domain and process (2nd ed.). *American Journal of Occupational Therapy, 62*(6), 625-683.)

Leisure

Leisure activities are those intrinsically rewarding things one does when not obligated to be doing anything else. Leisure is a very important area of occupation, particularly for older people. Leisure is generally considered as activities that enhance one's quality of life, and is not usually regarded as being reimbursable goals. However, the performance skills and patterns required to perform leisure activities are transferable to a variety of occupations that are reimbursable. Therefore, leisure is usually approached indirectly in documentation, with a focus on functional performance skills and patterns. However, in some practice settings such as mental health, it might be appropriate to have leisure-related goals addressing coping mechanisms, appropriate use of leisure time, or interpersonal or social components.

Play

In a young child, play can be solitary or social and may consist of organized tasks such as games with rules, or spontaneous activities such as exploratory play. One of the primary occupations for a child is acquiring those skills necessary to progress through age-appropriate developmental milestones, and these skills are acquired through play. When providing occupational therapy to young children, you will often find yourself talking about play in your documentation.

Education

Education is another of the primary occupations of a child. Those activities and skills needed to perform well in formal or informal educational settings are unique. Occupational therapy services to children in the educational system are for the purpose of the child successfully performing school-related activities. If you are working in school-based practice, your goals and interventions must relate to behaviors and skills needed in the classroom or school environment to be reimbursable. You should also consider the child's ability to engage in extracurricular activities such as music, clubs, and sports. Education for adults encompasses college classes and formal, informal, or personal educational situations such as attending a continuing education seminar for professional needs or personal enrichment (AOTA, 2008b).

Social Participation

People, as social beings, need to be able to interact successfully with others and to keep one's behavior within the contextual norms of the community, the family, and peer groups. If you are working with clients who have brain injury, developmental disability, or mental health conditions, you might find yourself documenting goals and interventions for social participation.

Rest and Sleep

Proper rest, relaxation, and sleep are essential for physical and emotional health, stamina, and safety. Clients who have pain, illness, or incontinence, or who are caregivers of young children or a parent with Alzheimer's disease may have interrupted sleep patterns or limited opportunities to rest or relax. Mental health conditions such as depression or anxiety can result in excessive or inadequate sleep. Other factors such as working multiple jobs or a noisy environment will also impact proper rest and sleep. Your documentation should include any concerns related to sleep preparedness or inadequate rest and sleep patterns.

Roles of the Occupational Therapist and Occupational Therapy Assistant

OTs and OTAs have different roles and responsibilities in documenting the occupational therapy intervention process. In AOTA's *Guidelines for Supervision, Roles, and Responsibilities During the Delivery of Occupational Therapy Services* (AOTA, 2009) and *Standards of Practice for Occupational Therapy* (AOTA, 2010c), the roles and responsibilities of both OTs and OTAs are very specifically delineated regarding documentation and clinical practice. The OTA partners with the supervising OT in designing, implementing, and assessing occupational therapy services (AOTA, 2009, 2010c). The OTA may also contribute to documentation at all stages of treatment under the supervision of the OT and concurring with relevant laws and regulations (AOTA, 2009, 2010c).

Although these guidelines are considered "best practice," state statutes and licensure laws may differ from the guidelines. The guidelines may also differ from federal laws that delineate mandatory documentation requirements. In addition, funding sources may specify who would be an approved documenter or service provider for reimbursement purposes. You, as an occupational therapy professional, are accountable for adhering to the mandatory policies and procedures adopted by state and federal regulatory agencies. However, you will find the standards established by AOTA very useful in interpreting and following regulations.

Types of Notes

Different kinds of notes are written at different stages of the occupational therapy process. Notes also vary according to the type of practice setting. From the first notation in the chart that a referral has been received to the closing lines of the discharge report, occupational therapy practitioners document the many varied activities of the intervention process. The specific content of the note, format and organization of the note, and the timelines required all vary according to type of setting, accrediting and regulatory agencies involved, and requirements of the funding source. The contents required for the following types of note are described in *Guidelines for Documentation of Occupational Therapy* (AOTA, 2008a) and will be addressed in this manual.

Initial Evaluation Reports

Before beginning treatment, the client is evaluated to determine whether occupational therapy is appropriate for this client, and if so, what kind of therapeutic intervention will be most useful. The OT directs the initial evaluation process, documents the results, and establishes the intervention plan, although the OTA can contribute to this process (AOTA, 2009, 2010c). Each practice setting or facility has its own way of evaluating a client. A behavioral or mental health center, for example, may not do the same kind of an initial evaluation as a public school or a skilled nursing facility. Initial evaluations are usually documented on specific forms provided by the setting but may also be done in a SOAP format.

Contact Notes

Each time an intervention is provided by the occupational therapy practitioner, a notation is made of what occurred. Contacts may also include pertinent telephone conversations and meetings with the client, family/caregiver, other professionals, or service providers (AOTA, 2008a). Depending on the setting, each treatment session is documented in the health or school record using a formal contact note or, perhaps, the occupational therapy practitioner might simply fill out a flow sheet or checklist of services provided. In other settings, the occupational therapy practitioner might only keep an attendance sheet or informal log or make notes to himself for use later in writing progress notes, but no formalized contact note is required. Contact notes can be written in many different formats, but in this manual the SOAP format will be taught.

Progress Report

At the end of a specified period of time, a progress note is written. The occupational therapy practitioner records the client's progress toward goals and details any changes made in the intervention plan. Different practice settings vary regarding time periods for reporting, but progress notes are usually written weekly, biweekly, or monthly. Progress notes may also be written in different formats, but will be taught in a SOAP format in this manual.

Reevaluation Report

The OT directs and documents the reevaluation that is part of the occupational therapy intervention process and modifies the intervention plan according to the client's needs. The OTA may contribute to this reevaluation process (AOTA, 2009, 2010c). Some settings require a formal reevaluation report. For example, in a practice setting where managed care is involved, a client may need to be reevaluated in order to be recertified for treatment after the number of initially allocated visits are completed.

Transition Plan

Transition notes are written when a client is transferring from one service setting to another (such as from early intervention to preschool or from special education to vocational services) within the same system of service delivery (AOTA, 2008a). Transition notes ensure that the client's intervention plan remains intact through the move and that services that have already been provided are not duplicated. The transition plan is the responsibility of the OT, but the OTA may contribute to this process (AOTA, 2009, 2010c).

Discharge or Discontinuation Report

At the end of treatment, a discharge or discontinuation report is written to describe changes in the client's ability to engage in meaningful occupation as a result of occupational therapy intervention (AOTA, 2008a). The discontinuation plan is directed and documented by the OT, but the OTA may contribute to this process (AOTA, 2009, 2010c). Discharge notes summarize the course of treatment; progress toward goals; status at the time of discharge; provision or recommendation of any durable medical equipment, adaptive devices, splints, or home programs; and any other referrals or follow-up required. Some settings will provide a specific form for the discharge note. Other facilities may use the same form that was used for the client's evaluation.

Names, demographic information, and other details have been eliminated or changed in this manual due to space limitations and to protect the confidentiality of those people who receive our services. If you were writing an actual note in a client's health record, you would use the client's whole name and any other required identifying information. In addition, all notes must be signed with the occupational therapy practitioner's full name and credentials. You should also realize that each client has unique circumstances and needs. Although this manual provides sound guidelines for documenting occupational therapy practice, you must always use your clinical judgment when treating clients and documenting in the record.

Conclusion

The following two worksheets will help you practice using the *Framework-II* terminology to record your observations. Then, in the following chapters, you will be introduced to the health record and to the specifics of your documentation in the record. Professional documentation pulls together all of your observation skills, clinical reasoning, and knowledge of occupational therapy. There will be ample explanation and opportunity for practice so that you will systematically acquire the appropriate documentation skills. Eventually, **you** will be the OTA we talked about in the beginning paragraph whose documentation was so amazing to the beginning student.

Worksheet 1-1
Using the *Occupational Therapy Practice Framework*

Observe someone make an object out of clay or another craft project. Use terminology from the *Occupational Therapy Practice Framework: Domain and Process, 2nd Edition* and list 10 specific performance skills or client factors that you observe or assess during this activity. Try to describe, qualify, or quantify levels of performance.

Activity Observed: _____

Examples:

    Performance skill: Cognitive—attends well to task

    Client factor: Has good range of motion in both hands

1.

2.

3.

4.

5.

6.

7.

8.

9.

10.

Morreale, M. J., & Borcherding, S. (2013). *The OTA's guide to documentation: Writing SOAP notes (3rd ed.).* Thorofare, NJ: SLACK Incorporated.

Worksheet 1-2
Occupational Therapy Practice Framework—More Practice

Observe someone perform a cooking task such as making tea, a sandwich, or can of soup. Use terminology from the *Occupational Therapy Practice Framework: Domain and Process, 2nd Edition* and list 10 specific performance skills or client factors that you observe or assess during this activity. Try to describe, qualify, or quantify levels of performance.

Activity Observed: _____

Example:

Motor and praxis skill: Coordinates use of both hands well when using can opener

Client factor: Able to hear whistling tea kettle

1.

2.

3.

4.

5.

6.

7.

8.

9.

10.

Morreale, M. J., & Borcherding, S. (2013). *The OTA's guide to documentation: Writing SOAP notes (3rd ed.).* Thorofare, NJ: SLACK Incorporated.

Chapter 2

The Health Record

Definition and Purpose

The "medical record" is now referred to as the "health record." It is a **legal document** that provides a written history of a client's past and present health, substantiates care, and creates proof of advance directives, vital statistics, course of treatment, and related correspondence (Fremgen, 2009; Scott, 2013). The primary purpose of the health record is the exchange of information among health care providers in order to determine a client's problems and strengths, develop an appropriate plan, record treatment, facilitate continuity of care upon discharge (or in the future), and fulfill legal documentation requirements (Fremgen, 2009; Scott, 2013). Besides an individual's health care information, records typically contain standard content such as the person's identifying information, demographic data, contact information, insurance and physician information, assignment of benefits, privacy notices, and consent forms. Occupational therapy practitioners in inpatient, outpatient, and community settings will use the health record frequently to obtain and document essential client information for care and reimbursement.

OTs and OTAs working in school-based settings provide interventions and documentation that focus primarily on the educational needs of children requiring special services. It is important to understand that a student's **education records** (including any occupational therapy documentation) also require accurate recordkeeping, confidentiality, and adherence to protocols. Education records provide a means of communication among professionals in the child's school and district concerning the child's academic abilities and pertinent medical or social concerns. Education records are also used to obtain aggregate data for local, state, and federal reports. While this manual often refers to the "health record," many of the documentation "rules" also apply to education records. Specific information regarding occupational therapy documentation in school-based settings is presented in Chapter 17.

A profession called *Health Information Management* was created to oversee the health record. The American Health Information Management Association (AHIMA) at www.ahima.org offers useful resources regarding various aspects of the record. As we move further into the information age, the health record continues to change rapidly. As medicine advanced, so did the complexity and detail of the health record. There has been an increasing shift toward the use of a computerized format, called an *electronic health record* (EHR) or *electronic medical record* (EMR), to manage and store client information. The Centers for Medicare and Medicaid Services (CMS) even initiated ongoing incentive programs in 2011 to provide eligible health professionals and hospitals with monetary incentives to adopt and use EHR technology meaningfully, such as reporting clinical quality measures (CMS, 2012b).

Electronic records are maintained by the provider. However, there are many different software programs and systems available, depending on the type of practice setting and funding source. For example, providers who are reimbursed by Medicare and Medicaid must use **certified** EHR technology in order to meet specific requirements for security and functionality (CMS, 2012b). Another type of computerized record, called a *personal health record*

Morreale MJ, Borcherding S.
The OTA's Guide to Documentation:
Writing SOAP Notes, Third Edition (pp 11-22).
© 2013 SLACK Incorporated.

(PHR), is a more recent trend (Gateley & Borcherding, 2012). A PHR is an EHR used and controlled by the individual rather than a provider or facility, thereby allowing individuals to maintain and organize their own health information for personal/family use or to selectively share with health care providers (CMS, 2012g). Your facility will provide training for whatever computerized or paper-based documentation system is in place there.

Electronic Documentation

As previously noted, advances in technology have created widespread use of computerized health care information systems. Many facilities have switched to paperless systems for documentation and reimbursement, thereby changing how occupational therapy practitioners approach the documentation process, use specific formats, communicate with others, and bill for services. Information can now be entered and obtained from different locations and means such as handheld wireless devices, desktop and laptop computers, telephones, and the Internet.

EHRs help standardize, streamline, and organize information, thus improving efficiency and decreasing the need for storage space (Herbold, 2010). Documentation completed using paper and pen often necessitates that health care providers fill out duplicate information (particularly client identifiers and demographic data) on facility and regulatory forms; this redundancy is minimized with EHR (Herbold, 2010). Another benefit of computerized (electronic) documentation is that it typically includes the use of prompts or check-offs for information necessary to meet requirements for the setting or funding sources (Pierson & Fairchild, 2008). Additionally, computerized documentation helps facilitate reporting outcome measures used in different settings, such as the Minimum Data Set (MDS) or Functional Independence Measure (FIM) (Herbold, 2010). Computerized documentation allows people in different departments or facilities to send and receive information easily and in a timely manner. Several people can review client data at the same time, such as medical orders, lab results, or clinical assessments from other disciplines. This can help to coordinate care and reduce duplication of tests or procedures. However, reasonable safeguards must be put in place to protect client privacy (U.S. Department of Health and Human Services [USDHHS], 2002, 2009). For example, health care workers typically have password-protected computer access to information needed to perform their job functions and must be educated regarding proper protection and disposal of client files (USDHHS, 2002, 2009).

Staff must be trained in the use of a particular software program or system. This could be time consuming or meet resistance from staff inexperienced with computers or used to documenting "the old way." When learning a new system, practitioners may experience an adjustment period requiring additional documentation time to merge their own organizational style with a more structured format. Depending on the setting, the OTA might share a computer in the occupational therapy office, enter data in a more central area, or have a personal laptop or digital device to access and record information. EHRs do create significant concerns regarding security, privacy, computer downtime, and "crashing." Also, information might be accidentally destroyed or entered inaccurately due to errors in typing, using a touch screen, or clicking a mouse. Another concern is that devices containing sensitive information on hard drives or discs could be stolen or lost.

There are many products and software programs available for evaluations, clinical notes, care plans, home exercise programs, and departmental tasks. Examples of therapy software and video demonstrations can be found using an Internet search engine. In clinical practice, occupational therapy practitioners might use electronic technology for various functions, such as the following:

- Organizing and managing a schedule
- Developing forms
- Tracking productivity
- Billing and reimbursement
- Completing required facility/agency instructional modules (e.g., infection control, sexual harassment, privacy laws)
- Continuing education
- Research
- Networking through professional organizations and social media
- Communicating with physicians, other disciplines, clients, or third-party payers
- Sending and receiving documents

- Receiving or requesting orders for occupational therapy
- Reviewing health records
- Recording data and assessment results
- Documenting all stages of the intervention process
- Utilizing and documenting clinical pathways
- Using outcomes measures
- Selecting from a standard word bank or menu of problems, goals, and possible intervention strategies specific to a particular practice setting
- Developing instructional materials/home programs for clients

OTs and OTAs must always use clinical reasoning and a client-centered approach throughout the occupational therapy process, including the recording of client data, developing goals, choosing interventions, or creating home programs. The terminology or methods used in a facility's software program may not be fully compatible with occupational therapy language or departmental needs. Therefore, occupational therapy practitioners must be careful to avoid a rote or cookbook approach when selecting problems, goals, and interventions from a computer program. Some software programs are very structured and rigid while others offer flexibility in terms of customizing formats to the specifications of a facility or department (such as for evaluations, treatment notes, and intervention plans). Some software programs allow for greater individualized detail by providing places for comments or allowing users to "mix and match" programs or menus. Practitioners must not lose sight of a client's individual needs or compromise quality care by making the client conform to the specifications of a particular software package. Additional information on computer generated plans is presented in Chapter 17.

Health Insurance Portability and Accountability Act

In 1996 Congress passed the Health Insurance Portability and Accountability Act (HIPAA), which established national standards to manage and protect the privacy and security of an individual's health information (USDHHS, 2003a). HIPAA delineates an individual's right to understand and control the use of one's own health information and also be informed about a provider's privacy practices, including how one's information will be used and shared (USDHHS, 2003a, 2003b).

The Privacy Rule required compliance by April 14, 2003 (with a 1-year extension for small health plans) (USDHHS, 2003a). It specified regulations for the use and disclosure of **protected health information** (PHI), which is defined as "individually identifiable health information" (USDHHS, 2003a, p. 3). Facilities and individuals providing health and medical services and transmitting health information electronically (i.e., claims, referral authorization requests, payment) are considered a **covered entity** (USDHHS, 2003a). Occupational therapy practitioners come under this category and must adhere to the HIPAA regulations.

A major part of the Privacy Rule is the **minimum necessary** standard, which states that only the minimum amount of protected health information must be requested or disclosed to accomplish the intended purpose (USDHHS, 2002, 2003a, 2003b). In addition, the covered entity must establish reasonable safeguards, workplace policies and procedures protecting PHI, such as limiting access only to personnel requiring information for their job duties and locking up records (USDHHS, 2002, 2003b). Some instances in which PHI disclosure is permitted without express written authorization include public health activities (e.g., tracking certain communicable diseases or adverse effects of products), various law enforcement situations, organ and tissue donation, reports of child abuse or neglect, and national security (USDHHS, 2003a).

In practical terms, as an OTA, you typically cannot provide information about the client's condition with the client's family, friends, or employer without the client's permission. However, you can usually communicate with the referring physician and other team members involved in the client's care. Also, although you might be very curious and concerned, those are not acceptable reasons to look up information on a friend, colleague, or family member who was admitted to the facility. Most importantly, you must always try to protect client privacy and safeguard information. As this is only a brief overview of HIPAA, **it is essential that you do not disclose or give out any health records or client information without fully understanding the law and knowing your facility's policies and procedures.**

Family Educational Rights and Privacy Act

The Family Educational Rights and Privacy Act (FERPA) outlines a student's rights and privacy regarding his or her education records (U.S. Department of Education, 2011). This federal law allows the parent or eligible student (i.e., students 18 or older or who attend schools beyond high school) to fully review the student's education record and to formally request correction of any inaccuracies, including what is written in occupational therapy (U.S. Department of Education, 2011). FERPA also mandates that, in order for a school to release a student's protected information, written permission from a parent or eligible student is needed (U.S. Department of Education, 2011). There are some exceptions for the consent requirement such as for emergencies, a student's financial aid, judicial orders, legitimate functions of school officials, and more (U.S. Department of Education, 2011). Schools are also allowed to release basic directory information (e.g., names, awards, honors) as long as parents are notified of this general practice and can opt out (U.S. Department of Education, 2011). If you are an OTA working in a school-related setting, it is essential that you do not disclose or give out any student records without fully understanding the law and knowing your school district or facility policies and procedures.

Storing, Managing, and Retaining Health Records

There are federal and state guidelines for storing, managing, and retaining health records. Each facility establishes its own policies and procedures to comply with this process, and the OTA must follow these protocols. The health record is the physical property of the health care facility that furnishes the client's care, but clients do have a legal right to obtain and review copies of their health information, including what you have written in occupational therapy (Fremgen, 2009; Scott, 2013). In order to obtain their records, clients usually have to write a formal signed request and may also be charged for the copying costs. Your facility will have specific policies regarding this process.

Third-party payers may require health record documentation to substantiate claims for reimbursement. In those cases, generally the original paperwork stays in the chart and copies are sent electronically, mailed, or faxed as appropriate to the situation. In some instances, occupational therapy documentation might require a physician signature such as to follow through with verbal orders or to certify for Medicare that an outpatient requires skilled services and the physician approves the plan of care. As previously mentioned, **privacy laws regulate the disclosure of medical information, so never, ever, give out or send any health records or client information without knowing the exact policies and procedures in your facility**. Each facility establishes a system to comply with laws, payer requirements, and to delineate which departments or personnel (e.g., Health Information Services Department or the outpatient department secretary) are responsible for sending out specific records or reports to clients, physicians, other professionals, or funding sources, depending on the situation. All staff must be very careful when using fax machines, copiers, and e-mail to avoid breaches of confidentiality to unintended recipients. Paperwork must be removed after using the copier, printer, or fax machine and it is prudent for the sender to always double check fax numbers and e-mail addresses for accuracy. A copy of pertinent correspondence, including letters, home exercise programs, or instructions, should be maintained in the record.

Active client charts may be held in a school or agency's administrative office, be held at a facility's central location (e.g., nurse's station), or stay within each discipline's department, such as within outpatient occupational or physical therapy departments (Sames, 2010). In facilities where records are normally held at the nurse's station, records may proceed with the client to other areas of the facility, such as the radiology department or occupational therapy room (Sames, 2010). Records should remain and be completed on-site and not taken home to review or complete documentation. However, an occupational therapy practitioner working in home care or traveling among several sites might have access to electronic records off-site or be allowed to keep a temporary working copy of records while the original stays within the agency. Again, it is essential to always follow HIPAA guidelines and facility policies.

To ensure privacy of a client's active or inactive health or education information, keep records in a secure location such as a locked file cabinet, drawer, storage unit, or office rather than leaving them open on your desk, treatment table, or mat or visible on a computer screen where they might inadvertently be seen by others (Sames, 2010). When using electronic records, be sure to properly log out or close the computer screen after looking at or recording client information, particularly if you share a computer or office with other staff. Volunteers, visitors, or other employees such as housekeeping, maintenance, secretaries, or other disciplines may have valid reasons to enter your office or treatment area, so you should manage records properly at all times to protect confidentiality. In addition, be especially careful when you are entering information or conversing about clients during a treatment session or in public areas. You must ensure that other people cannot inappropriately see or hear the confidential information.

Records may be stored in their original paper format or on microfilm, hard drives, or computer disks, depending on federal and state regulations and the type of practice setting (Scott, 2013). Individual states mandate the specific minimum time periods for retaining medical records for minors and adults, including occupational therapy documentation. Most states require that the health records of minors be kept until a certain number of years after the child reaches the age of majority in that state (Scott, 2013). Records may be kept longer than the state minimums for various reasons, such as possible future care of the client or tort concerns (Scott, 2013). It is essential that records that are no longer needed are destroyed properly (e.g., incineration or shredding) rather than just thrown into a garbage pail, so that no one else can ever read the confidential health information (Sames, 2010; USDHHS, 2009). Realize that any other paperwork or electronic files containing confidential client information not normally kept in the chart (such as any personal notations, drafts, or working copies used for day-to-day occupational therapy treatment), must also be properly secured and later destroyed. Most departments have shredders or designated locked bins readily available for proper disposal of confidential information.

SOAP Note History

In the 1960s, Dr. Lawrence Weed advocated the problem-oriented medical record (POMR) in order to provide a more structured and client-centered approach to the medical record (Pierson & Fairchild, 2008; Quinn & Gordon, 2010). The problem-oriented medical record consists of four components (Pierson & Fairchild, 2008):

1. A data base (e.g., client's history, physical evaluations by all disciplines, lab results)
2. A list of the client's current problems
3. An interdisciplinary treatment plan
4. Progress notes delineating treatment and status updates regarding specific problems

Weed recommended that the progress note include the client's own perception of the situation, which had previously been considered irrelevant. He organized the progress note into four distinct sections and called it a SOAP note (Pierson & Fairchild, 2008; Quinn & Gordon, 2010). The acronym SOAP stands for subjective, objective, assessment, and plan and consists of the following:

- **S (Subjective)**: The *client's perception* of the treatment being received, progress, limitations, needs, and problems. Normally the subjective section of a treatment note is brief. However, in an occupational therapy initial evaluation note, the "S" might be longer because it contains the information obtained by occupational therapy practitioners in the initial interview

- **O (Objective)**: The *health professional's observations* of the treatment being provided, such as the specific interventions implemented, the client's performance, and levels of assistance needed. In an occupational therapy initial evaluation note, this section also contains all of the measurable, quantifiable, and observable data that the OT determines should be collected. In an evaluation, the first two sections form the data base from which the OT, with contributions from the OTA, develops a problem list and treatment plan.

- **A (Assessment)**: The *health professional's clinical judgment and interpretation* of the statements and events reported in the subjective and objective sections. This section includes the client's progress, functional limitations, problems, and expectations of the client's ability to benefit from therapy (sometimes called *rehabilitation potential*). In an initial evaluation, the OT, with feedback from the OTA, will determine and include the problem list, which is one of the key elements of the POMR method of charting.

- **P (Plan)**: *What the health professional plans to do next* to help meet the goals and objectives in the intervention plan. In an occupational therapy initial evaluation, this section contains the OT's intervention plan, including the anticipated frequency and duration of treatment.

The POMR is not as popular now, although the SOAP note component has remained in common practice. Many facilities utilize a format called the **source-oriented medical record** to organize all of the client's health information in the chart. A source-oriented record is divided into sections for each discipline (i.e., nursing, lab results, occupational therapy, etc). Within each section, the discipline's information is presented in chronological order using SOAP notes (or another format) to record that discipline's care and the client's status. This type of organization makes it easy to locate information or track progress for a particular discipline such as occupational therapy. This is especially beneficial when contributing to an occupational therapy progress report or discharge report. A disadvantage is that one has to search through many sections to determine the client's overall status at a given time.

Another format used in some settings is the **integrated medical record**. With this format, all disciplines record information in chronological order, one right after the other. For example, an occupational therapy note might come directly after a nursing note, followed by a physical therapy note or respiratory therapy note. While this format makes it easy to find client information pertaining to a particular time period, it is harder to find or track information for a particular discipline. The OTA must search through all of the shift changes of nursing notes to find out what was done in the client's occupational therapy session yesterday. It is also more difficult to locate and gather information for the occupational therapy discharge report, such as the number of sessions provided.

All health record documentation must be in accordance with facility policies and legal and ethical standards. SOAP is simply a format—an outline for organizing information. Any note can be written in this format, although some notes lend themselves to it better than others. OTs and OTAs often use the SOAP format for contact (treatment) notes and progress notes to record client care and to document progress toward goals. The SOAP format forces the writer to look at all four aspects of the intervention session and to present the information contained in the note in a standard, organized way. A more detailed discussion of each section of the SOAP note will follow in Chapters 6 through 10.

Narrative Notes

An alternative to the SOAP format is the **narrative note**. Narrative notes are typically written in a less restricted paragraph format, although the information may be organized into pertinent categories such as client factors or areas of occupation. As narrative notes are not divided into standard sections like the SOAP note, the occupational therapy practitioner must be very careful to ensure that all of the necessary information is still included. A good narrative note will contain all of the ordered components of the SOAP note but just not have the information divided into separate categories for the S, O, A, and P. The general documentation "rules" in this manual still apply to narrative notes, but you might find that the information typically presented in the S and O sections of the SOAP note might sometimes be written in reverse order in a narrative note. If you first learn the SOAP note format presented in this manual, you can easily convert your client information into a proper narrative note if that is the format your facility uses. An example of a narrative discharge report is provided in Chapter 16, and several examples of narrative contact notes are provided in Chapter 18.

Users and Uses of Health Records

The health record is a communication tool and, thus, has many different uses and users. As an OTA, it is important to consider all of your different audiences when you make an entry in the client's record.

Client Care Management

The record is one method the treatment team uses to communicate with each other about the day-to-day aspects of a client's care. Other occupational therapy practitioners in your department or other members of the treatment team will read your notes in order to coordinate care. The OT, with contributions from the OTA, will document the results of the occupational therapy evaluation in the health record and establish the intervention plan. The OT and OTA will then collaborate to implement treatment, record the client's progress toward established goals, and advise other team members of the occupational therapy plan for continuing care. This communication is extremely important to the treatment team. One occupational therapy practitioner may not be providing all of the client's care and may depend upon the treatment notes to find out what treatment was provided in his or her absence.

Reimbursement

The record is the source document for what services were provided, and thus, for what occupational therapy services may be billed. It is used in billing to substantiate reimbursement claims. For example, if a question arises about the duration and frequency of interventions provided, the record would be the source document used to answer that question. Often in managed care, initial evaluation data and periodic progress reports must be submitted in order to obtain pre-authorization for subsequent therapy sessions.

The Legal System

The health record is a legal document that substantiates what occurred during a client's illness or condition and course of treatment. If you as an OTA have to appear in court to testify, you will be very glad that your documentation is clear and thorough. Sometimes court cases will occur years after the event or intervention that is being contested and you may not even remember the client or the event. What you have written in the record should provide you with the information you need to testify. Therapy records may be subpoenaed for many reasons, including cases involving Workers' Compensation, malpractice, personal injury lawsuits, child abuse, spousal abuse, or elder abuse.

Research and Evidence-Based Practice

The record is also used to provide data for medical research and evidence-based practice. Researchers might use individual data specific to that client or aggregate data where no client name is attached to the data. In either case, the source document is often the health record, under the security regulations of HIPAA.

Accreditation

Accrediting organizations, such as the Joint Commission and the Commission on Accreditation of Rehabilitation Facilities (CARF), review medical records (including your occupational therapy notes) to help ascertain whether the extent and quality of services provided by your facility and/or your department meet the standards of care set by the accrediting agency. If the facility is found not in compliance, accreditation may be withdrawn. Accreditation from certain national accrediting organizations, such as the Joint Commission, can be used to meet Medicare certification requirements for facilities and providers that bill Medicare (CMS, 2012a). If the facility or equipment provider does not meet CMS standards, claims made by that facility for Medicare services (including occupational therapy) will be denied. The health record is one of the primary sources used during a visit from an accrediting organization or a CMS State Survey Agency.

Education

The record may be used as a teaching tool. A student uses the health record to gain information about clients and learn about quality and appropriate occupational therapy intervention, in accordance with HIPAA guidelines.

Public Health

The health record is used to identify and to document the incidence of certain diseases, such as tuberculosis or HIV and outbreaks of contagious illness within a facility. In addition, the health record is used to report vital statistics (births, deaths); substantiate and report child, spousal, or elder abuse; and provide statistics for epidemiology.

Business Development

Management teams use the information contained in the record to review what kinds of clients are being seen and how services in the facility are being utilized. This information is used to help plan and market the services provided and to determine appropriate levels of personnel. For example, are enough cases of clients with cardiac conditions being admitted to open a specialized cardiac rehabilitation program? Would this necessitate hiring more staff in the occupational or physical therapy departments?

The Client

Another significant user is the client himself. When you are writing in the record, always remember that the client (or parent/guardian) has access to the information in his or her own health or education record and may choose to exercise his or her right to read what you have written.

Documentation for Quality Improvement

Many facilities have a Quality Improvement (QI) Committee whose duty it is to oversee the appropriateness and adequacy of the care that is being provided. This committee is in charge of finding and solving problems in client care. The health record is one of the primary sources of information used in the QI process. For example, the occupational therapy staff might determine that one problem they are seeing is that a certain percentage of outpatients are not complying with their splint-wearing schedule. The QI team collaborates with the occupational therapy department to brainstorm possible solutions and implement new procedures (e.g., providing clients with written instructions, reminder phone calls, or next day follow-up appointments) to address this problem. The occupational therapy practitioners will then document and track whether those new methods increase compliance.

Facilities also use other types of quality measures to determine if policies and procedures are being followed and to help ensure proper standards. One method is through the use of periodic **peer reviews**. Health professionals may be assigned various client records to review peer documentation and look for any deficiencies in notes or care implemented. For example, you might review another OTA's notes or another occupational therapy practitioner might review your notes for a client who has been discharged from therapy. Typically, the reviewer fills out a facility checklist or form as the chart is examined for predetermined criteria, such as if verbal orders have been followed up with a written order, all goals in the intervention plan have been addressed, or all the OTA's notes have been cosigned by the OT.

Following discharge from therapy or from the facility, clients may be asked to fill out a **client satisfaction survey**, which asks for the client's perspective about the care that was received from the facility, rehabilitation department as a whole, or a single discipline such as occupational therapy. These surveys are a useful tool for improving client care. In addition, positive reviews might also be a consideration used in incentive programs honoring deserving staff members.

Writing in the Record

Since health and education records are not only a communication tool during the client's course of treatment but also the source document for financial, legal, and clinical accountability, the record should indicate the following:

- What services were provided, where, and when
- What happened and what was said
- How the client responded to the service provided
- Why skilled occupational therapy services were needed rather than the services of an aide, teacher, or family member

Before you write anything in the record, make the following assumptions:

- Someone else will have to read and understand what I write because I may be sick or have the day off the next time this client needs to be treated.
- This entry I am about to make will be the one scrutinized by a CMS review team, Child Study Team, or managed care representative. If I were a funding source, would I want to pay for the occupational therapy services I am about to record?
- This entry I am about to make will be subpoenaed and scrutinized by attorneys. If I were called upon to testify, will I be able to recall pertinent client information based on this record?
- My client (or the client's parent/guardian) will exercise his or her right to read this record.

It is critical to know your payment sources when documenting. Payers have different requirements and time frames, and some look for quite different outcomes than others. With a client who has Medicare, you will normally discuss ADLs and write goals for self-care and home management as Medicare looks for **functional** improvement. It is not enough to simply indicate that the client is working toward a goal of increasing shoulder range of motion. You must indicate what this increased motion will enable the client to do, such as get food out of the refrigerator or put on a shirt. With a Workers' Compensation case, your documentation will be oriented toward the client's return to work or prevention of a costly injury. For example, a computer programmer who has carpal tunnel syndrome may benefit from ergonomic education, adaptive equipment, and a splint in order to alleviate symptoms for work tasks and prevent surgery. With home care, your documentation may focus on your client being unable to leave home to receive services or that you provided education to the caregiver regarding safety issues. If your documentation states that your client is shopping at the mall or driving to the grocery store, then payment will be denied as this indicates the client is not really homebound. For a child in Early Intervention, your notes will be oriented toward developmental needs, whereas for a school-age child, documentation will focus on educational performance as identified in the Individualized Education Program. Documentation for children in pediatric medical settings will focus on recovery or management of the child's medical condition to improve function and quality of life. Also remember the following facts when planning to write in the health record:

- Accuracy is your best protection against problems. You cannot be accurate if you wait too long to record what happened.
- A note in the health or education record will be a reflection of your professional identity and abilities as well as a reflection of your department and occupational therapy as a profession.
- No activity or contact is ever considered a service that has been provided until a clinical entry is in the record. In terms of legal and fiscal accountability, "If it is not written, it did not happen."

Here are some helpful hints on writing notes:
- Avoid generalities.
- Be as concise as possible without leaving out pertinent data.
- Report behavior objectively and avoid judgments except in assessing your data.
- Be sparse with technical jargon, which may be unfamiliar to the reader.
- Be careful when copying, typing, using touch screens, clicking a mouse, or writing down information to avoid errors.

The Mechanics of Documentation

There are "rules" that must be followed when writing in the health record:

1. **Use black ink that is waterproof and nonerasable.** Do not use a pencil or marker for notes entered into the record. Indelible ink will help ensure that notations are not altered or accidentally smeared (Gateley & Borcherding, 2012; Scott, 2013).

2. **Never use correction fluid or correction tape.** Using correction fluid or correction tape in a health record is considered illegally altering the record. Health records are legal documents that must always stand as originally written.

3. **Correct errors properly** (Fremgen, 2009; Kettenbach, 2009; Scott, 2013). If you make an error in the record, draw a single line through it, then date and initial your correction. Do not attempt to change a word or phrase by writing over it or squeezing in additional words.

   mm 3/15/13
   Pt. able to dress lower body with ~~verbal cues~~ min (A) using a reacher.

   Pt. able to dress lower body with ~~verbal cues~~ (mm 3/15/13) min (A) using a reacher.

   If you inadvertently write your note in the wrong client's chart, draw a single line through the entire entry and write "wrong chart" beside it with your signature and date.
   If you need to add something after you have written and signed your note, write an addendum with the current date and time.

4. **Do not erase.** This is also considered illegally altering the record and is another reason that indelible ink should be used.

5. **Do not leave blank spaces or lines.** Draw a horizontal line through the center of blank spaces. This prevents the record from being altered at a later date.

6. **Be sure all required data are present.** The *Guidelines for Documentation of Occupational Therapy* (AOTA, 2008a) specify requirements for each type of occupational therapy note such as an evaluation report, contact note, or discharge report. This information will be addressed in other chapters of this manual. Make certain that your documentation contains all of the required basic information such as the facility name, department name, and type of note (AOTA, 2008a). For source-oriented medical records, this is usually included as a heading at the top of each page and preprinted on your facility's forms (Figure 2-1). Your facility may also have different forms for each type of note. The following are some examples of headings:

XYZ Nursing Home
Occupational Therapy Department
Progress Note

XYZ Hospital
Occupational Therapy Department
___ Contact Note   ___ Progress Note   ___ Discharge Note

XYZ Home Health Care Agency
☐OT ☐PT ☐ST Department
Progress Note

The full name of your client must be included on each piece of documentation along with any applicable health record number or identification number (AOTA, 2008a). This will ensure that documentation is placed in the correct chart if papers accidentally get mixed up or if loose papers fall out of charts. Always check with your facility, but the client's name is generally written as last name, comma, then first name (Doe, Jane). Be especially careful to avoid clerical errors with record numbers, different spellings of similar sounding names (Jean, Gene, Jeanne), or unfamiliar or complex ethnic names (Coffman-Kadish, 2003).

7. **Sign and date every note.** Remember, it is absolutely critical that you date and sign all of your notes with your legal signature and credentials. **Do not** sign or enter information in the health record for someone else or ask someone to enter data for you (Pierson & Fairchild, 2008). Scott (2013) suggests that, in addition to a legible signature, a stamp printed with the health professional's legal name and credentials should be used near the signature. Notes written by an OTA and students may need a cosignature by a supervising OT when the agency, state, or federal regulations require this (AOTA, 2008a). In addition, some facilities require that you also document the time of day that occupational therapy services were provided or phone calls were made.

8. **Be concise.** In today's health care system, busy professionals are often pressed for time. They will appreciate being able to read what you have written in the shortest time possible, and your own time for documentation will also be limited under today's productivity standards.

9. **Use appropriate terminology for the recipients of services.** When referring to the persons who use occupational therapy services, terms such as *client, patient, consumer, resident, veteran, participant, individual, student, infant, child, caregiver,* or *family* may be used. Please use the term that is considered most respectful and appropriate for your practice setting.

10. **Be prudent in using abbreviations.** Use **only** the abbreviations that are approved by your facility and do not make up abbreviations. This will be further addressed in Chapter 4.

11. **Refer to yourself, the OTA, in the third person** (Kettenbach, 2009). Avoid referring to yourself with the words "I" or "me." For example, instead of recording, "*Child attempted to kick me,*" write, "*Child attempted to kick COTA.*" As another example, instead of writing, "*I instructed the client in dressing skills,*" write, "*COTA instructed the client in dressing skills.*" However, in this instance, it is even better to focus on the client rather than the health care practitioner in your note (Kettenbach, 2009), such as, "*Client was instructed in dressing skills.*"

12. **Use proper spelling and grammar.** Facilities have different styles of organizing and writing information. Some facilities will allow you to use sentence fragments or incomplete sentences, and you will notice this in some of the examples in this book. Other facilities may have a more formal style and may insist on complete sentences. Follow the style used in your particular facility and always use proper spelling and grammar. This will be addressed further in Chapter 5.

13. **Notes continued.** If your note for a particular entry does not fit on one page, at the end write "*(cont.)*." Then, on the next page that you resume writing the same note, write the date and "*(OT note cont.)*" on the first line.

14. **Always adhere to ethical and legal guidelines.** Keep abreast of laws, regulatory guidelines, facility policies, and AOTA's documents concerning both the delivery of occupational therapy services and documentation. This includes anti-discrimination and privacy laws, issues regarding billing and reimbursement, fraud and abuse, certification, continuing competency, supervision, scope of practice, and other pertinent issues.

15. **Always be truthful and objective.** The information you record should never be misleading, fabricated, or falsified (AOTA, 2010a). Don't guess at or embellish information; be careful to avoid personal complaints; and do not judge, criticize, or blame other employees in your note. Defamatory statements could potentially be considered libel (Kettenbach, 2009; Scott, 2013).

16. **Write legibly, type carefully, and enter all information accurately.** Pharmacists, therapists, and other health providers are sometimes unable to decipher prescriptions and medical documentation due to illegible handwriting. Remember that other professionals and insurance companies will be reading and reviewing your

occupational therapy notes. You will also be providing written home programs for clients and caregivers. Sloppy handwriting or data entry errors using a keyboard, touch screen, or mouse may result in serious inaccuracies or substandard work, or it may possibly harm the client. It is essential that your notes be understandable and accurate in order to communicate effectively and avoid serious errors.

17. **Use people first language.** Emphasize the person rather than the disability. For example, instead of writing, "*autistic child*" or "*total hip replacement client,*" it is better to say, "*child with autism*" or "*client who had total hip replacement surgery.*"

18. **The OTA should not be referred to as "*therapist.*"** There is a clear distinction between an OT and an OTA (AOTA, 2009, 2010c). The OTA should be referred to as an *occupational therapy assistant* or an *occupational therapy practitioner* rather than a *therapist.* Medicare regulations regarding occupational therapy also state that the words *therapist* and *clinician* apply only to the OT and are not appropriate terms for the OTA (CMS, 2008a, 2008d).

19. **Always review the client's chart and communicate with the client and team members as appropriate before beginning treatment.** It is important to determine if there have been any changes in the client's status or discharge plan or if new medical orders are in place. For example, the client may have developed complications or may be undergoing testing that necessitates fasting, bed rest, or measuring fluid intake and output.

20. **Don't assume you will find all of the information you need in the chart.** You must always use clinical reasoning and good communication skills to decipher and clarify information present in the chart and determine what information or medical orders might be missing or incomplete. If you are unsure of something regarding a client, discuss it with your supervising OT or other team members as appropriate. When in doubt, always err on the side of caution.

Your occupational therapy documentation serves many purposes. When writing in the record, all occupational therapy practitioners and students are obliged to adhere to professional, legal, and ethical standards (AOTA, 2008a, 2010a). Follow the guidelines listed in this chapter for the basic rules of documentation. The subsequent chapters and worksheets will then help you to develop effective communication skills and improve clinical reasoning for documentation. Remain patient, keep practicing, and remember that someday soon your SOAP notes will be an important component of your client's health or education record.

Healthy Hospital
Occupational Therapy Department
Contact Note

Name: _____   Record #: _____

Date/Time	

Figure 2-1. Example of a facility form.

Chapter 3

Billing and Reimbursement

This chapter discusses legal and ethical considerations for reimbursement, guidelines for documentation, funding sources, and proper use of billing codes. It is important to realize this manual contains information based on current practice guidelines and legislation at time of publication. Reimbursement criteria and documentation requirements often change based on new laws and changes in the health care environment.

Skilled Occupational Therapy

Throughout this documentation manual, occupational therapy service is described as *skilled occupational therapy.* This term originated in Medicare regulations, which define the difference between skilled and nonskilled services (Centers for Medicare and Medicaid Services [CMS], 2006a, 2011a). Because Medicare requirements are quite stringent, those guidelines are being followed in this manual to help ensure that your services will not be denied payment by any payer. **Skilled** services have specific criteria and are performed by **qualified professionals**, including OTs and OTAs under the OT's supervision (CMS, 2008a, 2008e). They require professional education, decision making, and highly complex competencies that have a well-defined knowledge base of human functioning and occupational performance. **Nonskilled** services are defined as those that are routine or maintenance types of therapy, both of which could be carried out by nonprofessional personnel or caregivers (CMS, 2006a, 2011a). This manual emphasizes the necessity of documenting your intervention as **skilled occupational therapy**. This means you must demonstrate the client's potential for functional improvement and safety, or that intervention is necessary for equipment recommendations, for establishment of an effective and safe maintenance program, or to address a specific medical need (CMS, 2006a, 2011a). These criteria justify the services of an OT or OTA.

Reasonable and Necessary Care

The frequency, duration, type, and amount of therapy services must be **reasonable and necessary** based on the client's condition, rehabilitation potential, complexity, and accepted standard practices (CMS, 2006a). Medicare and other payers do **not** reimburse for services considered nonskilled or unnecessary for the client's condition, or if there is no expectation that treatment will be effective (CMS, 2006a, 2011a). If your client has a chronic condition or terminal illness, you might only be reimbursed one or two sessions for positioning or exercise. In that situation, you are expected to develop the appropriate intervention or prevention program, with follow-up provided by nonskilled personnel or a family member (CMS, 2006a, 2011a). It is necessary for you to document in a way that differentiates

Morreale MJ, Borcherding S.
The OTA's Guide to Documentation: Writing SOAP Notes, Third Edition (pp 23-30).

your skill as an occupational therapy practitioner from that of nursing or other rehabilitation disciplines. It is also important to document objective, measurable information and to clearly indicate any progress the client is making toward improving his or her impairment and restoring the prior level of function (CMS, 2006a). Realize that billing for extra services the client really does not need, keeping a client on a program longer than necessary, or billing for services not provided are unethical and could lead to severe legal and professional consequences.

The occupational therapy practitioner should only bill for actual treatment time, not ancillary tasks such as preparing the treatment area, transporting the client, reviewing charts, documenting, allowing for client toilet breaks or rest periods, etc. (CMS, 2003e). However, if your time transporting the client is also used for a pertinent intervention outlined in the OT's intervention plan (such as skilled instruction in wheelchair mobility or cognitive skills such as safety, problem solving, or topographical orientation), that time might then be billable. If the client's intervention plan includes areas such as dressing and transfers, you might take the opportunity of the client's necessary toilet break to work on skilled toilet transfers, managing clothing, and safety.

Justification for Skilled Therapy

Proper wording is critical to justify continuing skilled occupational therapy and demonstrate the level of complexity or sophistication of the services you are providing. **Never embellish or fabricate information to substantiate treatment**. Documentation must also reflect the treatment appropriate to the individual's condition and rehabilitation potential. The occupational therapy practitioner **provides skilled instruction** to clients rather than **assisting** them. For example, an occupational therapy practitioner may provide instruction in methods of energy conservation and work simplification rather than help the client perform a strenuous task. OTs and OTAs collaborate to **design** and provide **instruction** in home programs, which will then be carried out by aides, caregivers, and family members. Why should a third-party payer reimburse you to watch a client carry out the home exercise program that he performs daily on his own? However, if you are **assessing** the client's ability to do all of the components of it correctly, or **modifying** it to compensate for recent progress or changes, then your professional skill as an OTA is clearly required, under the supervision of the OT.

Consider the following specialized skills and services that occupational therapy practitioners provide:

- **OTs, with contributions from the OTA, provide the following services** (AOTA, 2009, 2010c):
  - Evaluate and reevaluate clients; identify problems; establish goals; and develop intervention, transition, and discontinuation plans
  - Assess or reassess the effectiveness of adaptive equipment, compensatory techniques, and therapeutic activities in order to modify the intervention plan for appropriate outcomes

- **OTs and OTAs provide the following services** (AOTA, 2008c, 2010b):
  - Modify and adapt activities, functional tasks, and environmental contexts such as workstations, classrooms, and homes to enable occupational performance
  - Modify activities through the provision, instruction, and use of adaptive equipment/assistive devices/ technology
  - Teach adaptive and compensatory techniques
  - Facilitate and improve developmental skills
  - Fabricate/modify/instruct in use of splints, orthotics, prosthetics, and adaptive devices
  - Provide individualized, specialized, and skilled instruction to the client/family/caregiver
  - Promote physical and psychosocial well-being
  - Determine the safety and effectiveness of performance skills, task procedures, and equipment
  - Intervene to address safety hazards and unsafe or at-risk behaviors
  - Improve performance skills and client factors through remediation approaches
  - Administer physical agent modalities as a means to facilitate occupational performance (AOTA, 2010b, 2012)

- **Specific types of skilled occupational therapy instruction to the client, family, or caregiver might include the following** (AOTA, 2008c, 2010b):
  o Instruction in individualized therapeutic exercise programs
  o Instruction in the development or remediation of specific life skills for occupational roles and contexts
  o Instruction in coping mechanisms, behavior management, and assertiveness training
  o Strategies for stress or anger management
  o Instruction in specific leisure, social, and interpersonal skills
  o Education regarding community services and support systems
  o Instruction in energy conservation and work simplification
  o Instruction in joint protection
  o Driver rehabilitation and education
  o Instruction in body mechanics, ergonomics, and functional mobility
  o Instruction in prevocational and vocational task skills
  o Education to promote health, wellness, safety, and life satisfaction
  o Instruction in positioning of the limbs, trunk, and head to facilitate ADLs and address client factors such as normalizing tone, reducing edema, and facilitating safe swallowing.
- **Skilled occupational therapy is NOT evident when the OT or OTA provides the following services** (CMS, 2006a, 2011a):
  o Provides unnecessary or unreasonable services for a client who cannot tolerate interventions, has poor potential to meet rehabilitation goals, or is expected to spontaneously recover a transient loss of function such as after a general surgery
  o Carries out diversionary activities or groups not appropriate or relevant to the intervention plan
  o Duplicates services with another discipline or provides services that nonskilled personnel are able to do
  o Continues routine interventions or maintenance programs such as self-care activities; passive range of motion; or monitoring of exercise programs after the adapted procedures are in place, outcomes are reached, or no further significant progress or changes are expected or needed
  o Provides services that are not part of an occupational therapy intervention plan
  o Has a patient watch a video or read a handout regarding total hip or cardiac precautions, home safety, ergonomics, body mechanics, etc., without providing skilled instruction or practice of the skills
  o Administers routine physical agent modalities without relating them to the performance of occupational tasks (AOTA, 2012)

Other Reimbursable Services

Safety Concerns

The ability to perform a task must include the ability to do it safely. Intervention strategies targeting safety are usually considered cost-effective services by third-party payers because they prevent costly reinjury. Safety concerns include situations such as a high probability of falling; lack of environmental awareness; severe pain; absent skin sensation; abnormal, aggressive, or maladaptive behaviors; or suicide risk. These all fall within the scope of skilled occupational therapy.

Prevention of Secondary Complications

Preventative interventions are within the scope of skilled occupational therapy if it can be shown that the client has a high risk of developing complications. Secondary complications might include prevention of repetitive strain injuries, progressive joint contractures, fracture nonunion, and skin breakdown or pressure sores. Other prevention programs and strategies might include early intervention programs, drug/alcohol relapse prevention programs, programs for at-risk youth, assessment of ergonomics in the workplace, instruction in joint protection, energy conservation, and provision of wellness programs.

Use of Aides

Many settings have nonprofessional staff such as OT aides, rehab aides, or technicians to assist with departmental tasks and improve productivity. It is important to realize that these are not licensed roles requiring professional education. Often, aides only receive on-the-job training. Functions of the aide may include clerical tasks (e.g., scheduling, photocopying, putting paperwork in charts); maintenance (e.g., laundry, cleaning equipment, keeping temperature logs, maintaining volume for superficial thermal modalities); and routine departmental tasks (e.g., servicing wheelchairs, organizing and ordering supplies, preparing areas for treatment, transporting clients, assisting the OT or OTA with a client in a group or during a transfer). According to AOTA's *Guidelines for Supervision, Roles, and Responsibilities During the Delivery of Occupational Therapy Services* (AOTA, 2009), **aides cannot provide skilled therapy**. They may be assigned client-related tasks only when the client outcome and environment are stable and predictable, professional judgment is not needed, and the task routine has already been established and performed by the client (AOTA, 2009). Additionally, the aide must be under the supervision of the occupational therapy practitioner and properly trained in the delegated tasks (AOTA, 2009). CMS regulations also clearly state that services provided by an aide are considered unskilled and, as such, are not a billable covered service, even under the supervision of an OT (CMS, 2006a, 2008e). Billing for services rendered by an aide as skilled procedures is unethical and could create legal and professional ramifications.

Funding Sources

While individuals can pay providers directly for health care services rendered, the majority of health care is funded through a wide range of public and private health insurance programs and managed care plans. Third-party payers vary greatly regarding program eligibility, premiums, out-of-pocket expenses, provider networks, and plan benefits such as preventative care, catastrophic care, and rehabilitation services.

An individual may purchase a private policy directly from an insurance company or might obtain insurance through one's own employer or an employer of a parent or spouse (Gateley & Borcherding, 2012). In some instances, private organizations and foundations may provide special grants to individuals to help pay for certain out-of–pocket health care costs such as therapy, medical equipment, or other services. Another reimbursement mechanism is **Workers' Compensation**, which is a mandatory insurance paid by businesses to cover employees who are injured on the job. Workers' Compensation pays for an injured employee's wages, medical care, and rehabilitation, although programs and benefits vary from state to state. A government-funded program called **TRICARE** provides health care services for active and retired military personnel and their families. **Medicare** and **Medicaid** are major public programs that provide health care benefits to eligible populations. Chapter 17 explains the Medicare and Medicaid documentation requirements for specific practice settings such as home care, acute care, outpatient, and skilled nursing facilities.

Medicare

Medicare is a federal insurance program for people 65 and older, individuals with end-stage renal disease, and eligible people younger than 65 who have permanent disabilities. The Medicare program obtains revenue through a designated Medicare payroll tax and consists of the following four parts (CMS, n.d.):

1. **Medicare Part A (Hospital Insurance):** This covers inpatient hospital care, limited skilled nursing facility stays, hospice, and some home health services. Premiums are generally free for individuals (and their spouse) if they paid Medicare taxes while working, but there are some expenses for care.

2. **Medicare Part B (Medical Insurance):** This is a supplemental insurance that generally covers outpatient care (such as occupational therapy), doctor's visits, preventative services, and medical supplies. Part B requires a monthly premium and there are some additional costs for care.

3. **Medicare Part C (Medicare Advantage Plans):** This is a type of Medicare plan that is contracted with private insurance companies to provide Medicare Part A and B benefits so costs vary. Plans usually include coverage for prescription drugs.

4. **Medicare Part D (Prescription Drug Coverage):** This provides prescription drug coverage through Medicare-approved companies, and costs vary.

Further information about Medicare eligibility, benefits, out-of-pocket costs, and plan limits can be found at www.medicare.gov.

Medicaid

Medicaid is a joint federal and state program that funds health care for eligible low-income people in the United States and its territories (CMS, 2012h). Medicaid covers more people and generates higher federal health care expenditures than Medicare (CMS, 2012h). Medicaid mandates coverage of certain health services but allows individual states flexibility to administer programs, determine other benefits, and process claims (CMS, 2012h). Therefore, eligibility, types of services covered, and reimbursement rates vary from state to state. Services may even be different for children than for adults within a particular state (Gateley & Borcherding, 2012). States often contract with managed care organizations to administer their Medicaid programs more effectively. OTs and OTAs must follow documentation and reimbursement guidelines for the state in which occupational therapy services are provided (Gateley & Borcherding, 2012). Further information about Medicaid and links to state programs can be found at www.medicaid.gov.

Early Intervention and Schools

Children less than 3 years of age who are experiencing a developmental delay (or are at risk for developmental delay due to a diagnosed condition) are eligible for **Early Intervention** services under Part C of the Individuals with Disabilities Education Act (IDEA) (Küpper, 2012). States have discretion to expand the definition of "at risk" factors to include environmental or biological factors and, if appropriate, may also extend a child's services until kindergarten (Küpper, 2012). The law mandates that early intervention services must be provided in the child's "natural environment," which can include the home or a community setting with typical children such as a daycare center or preschool (Küpper, 2012). IDEA Part B applies to children ages 3 to 21 with a disability, and the law requires that schools provide an appropriate free public education in the least restrictive environment (Gateley & Borcherding, 2012). Special education services, such as occupational therapy, may be provided to help the child succeed in school. The unique documentation requirements for school-based settings are described in Chapter 17.

Billing Codes

Diagnosis and billing codes are used by physicians and other health care providers when submitting claims for reimbursement. You, as an OTA, will need to assign the appropriate codes to your client's condition and interventions. Facilities establish specific procedures for the billing process and will provide you with the necessary resources. Code books may be purchased from various sources, and codes are also published on the CMS Web site.

Healthcare Common Procedure Coding System

The Centers for Medicare and Medicaid Services established the mandatory **Healthcare Common Procedure Coding System** (HCPCS) to enable physicians and other health care providers to use common language and standardized codes (CMS, 2009b, 2010a). These codes are used to identify and bill health services and medical products and to collect data. The system consists of two parts: Level I and Level II. Level I contains numerical codes called **Current Procedural Terminology** (CPT) codes that are maintained by the American Medical Association. These Level I codes are used to bill for individual procedures that the client receives, such as skilled therapy. Level II is maintained by CMS and consists of codes for health products such as durable medical equipment, prosthetics, orthotics, and supplies; chemotherapy drugs; and certain services not included in the Level I codes (American Academy of Professional Coders [AAPC], 2012b).

Inpatients with Medicare Part A benefits in settings such as hospitals and skilled nursing facilities come under the **prospective payment system**, which pays a predetermined Federal per-diem rate according to diagnoses and level of care needed (CMS, 2012e, 2012f). Therapy sessions are typically bundled into the daily rate rather than reimbursed separately. However, outpatient services or products that are covered under Medicare Part B benefits are generally reimbursed for each individual item according to the **Medicare Physician Fee Schedule** (MPFS) if all criteria are met (CMS, 2009b). Other payers establish their own criteria for reimbursement rates and what services are covered.

Medicare Physician Fee Schedule

Covered outpatient services and products are reimbursed according to current **established rates** in the MPFS (CMS, 2009b) as part of HCPCS. The health provider cannot be reimbursed more than the set rates even if the provider normally charges more for that procedure. The MPFS applies to a number of settings such as occupational therapy private practice, Comprehensive Outpatient Rehabilitation Facility, and some hospital and skilled nursing facility clients not covered with a Medicare Part A stay. (CMS, 2009b). Typically, funding sources require the client to pay a predetermined amount out-of-pocket, called a **deductible**, before the funding source will begin reimbursement. Some funding sources mandate that clients pay an out-of-pocket **copayment** amount (ranging from about $5.00 to $50.00) directly to the provider at each session. This copayment supplements what the funding source also pays the provider for that visit. For various commercial payers and Medicare, clients may be responsible for a **coinsurance** amount after meeting their deductible (CMS, 2003f, 2010c). Here is an example:

Occupational therapy procedure—$50.00 charged by occupational therapy clinic

Medicare allowable amount (MPFS)—$40.00

Medicare pays 80% of the $40.00, which equals $32.00

Patient is responsible for paying remaining 20% coinsurance of the $40.00, which equals $8.00.

Total reimbursement to occupational therapy clinic is $40.00 ($32.00 + $8.00)

Timed and Untimed Services

Some therapy codes are based on time using 15-minute intervals. Other therapy codes are considered untimed procedures and billed at a fixed amount (for that particular procedure) regardless of how much time is used (CMS, 2009a, 2011b). An occupational therapy evaluation (an untimed procedure) is only billed 1 unit regardless of how much time was needed or how many different assessment tools were used to complete the evaluation that day (CMS, 2009a, 2011b). Some codes are mutually exclusive and cannot be billed together (CMS, 2009a, 2011b). For example, codes requiring constant attendance or direct one-on-one patient contact (such as ADL instruction, ultrasound, or neuromuscular reeducation) cannot be billed together for one or two clients during the same 15-minute time period (CMS, 2009a, 2011b).

Medicare has very strict criteria regarding treatment rendered by therapy students. Those services require **appropriate supervision** by the qualified practitioner to qualify as a Part B skilled service; a supervisor's mere presence in the room is insufficient (CMS, 2006b, 2009a). Also, there are clear billing rules regarding treating more than one client at a time, which may require a cheaper group rate, or two disciplines performing a joint treatment to one client (CMS, 2006b, 2009a). If, for example, the OTA and PTA team up to perform a timed service for 30 minutes, those disciplines should divide the time in half and only bill 15 minutes each (CMS, 2009a). Realize that all timed services (e.g., therapeutic exercise, ADL instruction, wheelchair management training) are billed as 15-minute units but are actually considered by Medicare to be anywhere from 8 minutes to 22 minutes as per the following CMS chart (CMS, 2011b):

Units	Number of Minutes
1 unit:	≥8 minutes through 22 minutes
2 units:	≥23 minutes through 37 minutes
3 units:	≥38 minutes through 52 minutes
4 units:	≥53 minutes through 67 minutes
5 units:	≥68 minutes through 82 minutes
6 units:	≥83 minutes through 97 minutes
7 units:	≥98 minutes through 112 minutes
8 units:	≥113 minutes through 127 minutes, etc

Thus, if a client received skilled instruction and practice in transfers for 10 minutes and also worked on therapeutic exercise for 11 minutes, the total billable time would be 21 minutes, which equals only 1 billable unit. The service that consisted of the most time is billed, which is therapeutic exercise in this case. However, if the time spent on transfers was 10 minutes and therapeutic exercise was 25 minutes, total time equals 35 minutes, which is 2 units billed as 1 unit of each of the two services. Services cannot be billed if less than 8 minutes (CMS, 2011b).

To bill Medicare for therapy, a **claim form** called the CMS-1500 form is used by health providers and, in most cases, is submitted electronically (Fearon, Levine, & Quinn, 2010). Claims that are rejected due to clerical errors may be resubmitted with corrections. However, for fully denied claims or those reimbursed with reduced amounts, the provider might choose to go through an **appeals process** to substantiate the claim. There is also a mandated monetary limit for outpatient therapy services called a **therapy cap**, which specifies the maximum yearly amount that is reimbursable for a client with Medicare Part B (CMS, 2010b, 2010c). As this is just a brief overview of the billing process, it is imperative that occupational therapy practitioners be knowledgeable regarding current payer regulations.

ICD-9 and ICD-10 Codes

The World Health Organization (WHO) is responsible for the International Classification of Diseases (ICD). ICD is a large set of codes used to define and classify the spectrum of health-related conditions, injuries, disorders, and diseases worldwide (WHO, 2012a). ICD enables nations to track diseases and deaths (morbidity and mortality), manage health, and allocate resources (AAPC, 2012a; WHO, 2012a). ICD-9-CM refers to the 9th version of the ICD codes, which are currently in use in the United States (AAPC, 2012a). These codes are used for health care statistics and billing and are very specific in classification. For example, a fracture is coded by the particular bone, the part of bone, and whether it is a closed or open fracture. As of October 1, 2014, medical coders and billers in the United States will switch over to ICD-10-CM as mandated by the U.S. Department of Health and Human Services (AAPC, 2012a). The number of codes will dramatically increase from approximately 17,000 codes in ICD-9-CM to more than 141,000 codes in ICD-10, creating a transitional challenge (AACP, 2012a). Although ICD-10 has been in use worldwide since 1994, the United States is one of only several member countries that have not yet fully incorporated its use (AACP, 2012a). The WHO has already begun work on the next version, and it is expected that ICD-11 will be completed in 2015 (WHO, 2012a).

Helpful Resources for Billing and Reimbursement

The Medicare Learning Network, part of the CMS Web site (www.cms.gov), contains Web-based educational videos, fact sheets, and booklets regarding health benefits, documentation, billing, and reimbursement. Also, the CMS manuals can be accessed on the CMS Web site. Some sections applicable to occupational therapy include the following:

- Publication 100-02: Medicare Benefit Policy Manual
  - Chapter 7—Home Health Services [Section 40.2: Skilled Therapy Services]
  - Chapter 15—Covered Medical and Other Health Services [Section 220: Coverage of Outpatient Rehabilitation Therapy Services]
- Publication 100-04: Medicare Claims Processing Manual
  - Chapter 5—Part B Outpatient Rehabilitation [Sections 10, 20, 30]

The American Academy of Professional Coders Web site (www.aapc.com) has information and training materials regarding coding and billing. Another resource is the AOTA Web site (www.aota.org), which contains a section on reimbursement and regulatory policy and is a very useful resource to help determine what occupational therapy services are reimbursable. Information on early intervention and special education services can be found at the U.S. Department of Education Web site at www.ed.gov. Also, Chapter 17 in this manual explains the documentation criteria for reimbursement in different practice settings.

Worksheet 3-1
Use of Aides

Indicate which of the following tasks can be delegated to an occupational therapy aide by putting a YES (Y) or No (N) beside each of the following.

1. ___ Help maintain inventory of adaptive equipment and supplies.

2. ___ Place completed OT paperwork in medical charts.

3. ___ Instruct the client in new therapy putty exercises.

4. ___ Instruct the client in a sliding board transfer.

5. ___ Assist the OT practitioner with a client transfer.

6. ___ Upgrade a client's exercise program.

7. ___ Photocopy a home exercise program for the client's chart.

8. ___ Transport a stable client in a wheelchair from his hospital room to the OT room.

9. ___ While the OTA is leading a sensory group, assist a client in that group to handle tactile objects.

10. ___ Assist client in filling out client information forms.

11. ___ Teach a client how to use lower extremity adaptive equipment following a total hip replacement.

12. ___ Determine what adaptive feeding equipment is needed for a client who has a CVA with right hemiparesis.

13. ___ Schedule OT appointments.

14. ___ Select activities for a client's fine motor exercises.

15. ___ Assist the OTA with client wound care by opening bandage packages and instruments.

16. ___ Adjust settings on a TENS unit when client reports not feeling the treatment modality work.

17. ___ Sit and talk with a client while client is receiving a hot pack or other modality.

18. ___ Assist a child with scissors skills when more practice is needed after child learns the task and condition is stable.

19. ___ Obtain therapeutic equipment for the OTA to use with client.

20. ___ Cut out Velcro tabs and straps for a splint that OTA is fabricating.

21. ___ Administer part of a standardized assessment.

22. ___ Add more paraffin to unit when paraffin levels are low.

23. ___ Maintain temperature log of hydrocollator.

24. ___ Determine if a client should have a paraffin treatment rather than a hot pack that day.

25. ___ Set up client's meal tray in preparation for OT feeding session.

26. ___ Clean equipment and treatment tables/mats.

27. ___ Place reality orientation calendar in client's room.

28. ___ Determine if a client is adhering to weightbearing precautions during morning ADLs.

Chapter 4

Using Medical Terminology

Health care professionals are often pressed for time but are still obligated to complete documentation within established time frames. The use of symbols and abbreviations can certainly help to save time, but the OTA must use them very carefully and judiciously. Remember that your notes may be read by someone who knows little about occupational therapy and who will determine whether to pay for your services. In addition, other disciplines such as teachers, aides, or quality improvement personnel may not be familiar with certain medical jargon and may have difficulty interpreting the information. It is prudent to be sure that the person reading your notes is able to understand what you have written. Your facility will be able to furnish a list of the abbreviations it allows so that the abbreviations and symbols that you use will be validated if there is a question. **Do not make up your own abbreviations, and do not use any abbreviation that is not on your facility's approved list**. Remember that you are permitted to write out any word rather than shortening it or using a symbol. In this manual and in clinical practice, you will find that some settings or disciplines use more abbreviations and symbols than others.

The Joint Commission, which accredits hospitals and other health care facilities, does not maintain an approved list of acceptable abbreviations and symbols for use in documentation, but it does specify and update a list of those that are prohibited (Joint Commission, 2012). For example, the abbreviations QD (daily) and QOD (every other day) are prohibited because each can be easily mistaken as the other or confused with QID (four times a day) (Joint Commission, 2012). When in doubt, refer to the Joint Commission Web site at www.jointcommission.org. The Institute for Safe Medication Practices (ISMP) has compiled a larger list of abbreviations and symbols that are prone to error and miscommunication (ISMP, 2011). ISMP recommends that items on this list should never be used for medical communication such as written or verbal prescriptions, drug labels, or notations for medication administration (ISMP, 2011). This list can be referred to at the ISMP Web site (www.ismp.org).

In order to maintain uniformity and clarity in the health record, each health care facility establishes a list of approved abbreviations and symbols that may be used in documentation. An abbreviation may have more than one meaning so you must consider the context in which it is used. Consider the following statement:

> *Client needed HOH assist to hold the spoon and bring food to her mouth.*

As *HOH* is an abbreviation for "hard of hearing" and also "hand-over-hand," the only phrase that would make sense for that particular statement is:

> *Client needed **hand-over-hand** assist to hold the spoon and bring food to her mouth.*

It is also important to note that abbreviations are case sensitive, so you must always write them carefully. For example, *ADD* stands for "attention deficit disorder" yet *add* means "adduction." *PT* is "physical therapy" whereas *pt.* refers to "patient."

Morreale MJ, Borcherding S.
*The OTA's Guide to Documentation:
Writing SOAP Notes, Third Edition (pp 31-41).*
© 2013 SLACK Incorporated.

For purposes of using this manual, the following list of abbreviations in Table 4-1 will be permitted. Realize that this list is not all inclusive and that there are entire books devoted to medical abbreviations. As an OTA, you will certainly encounter many other commonly used and acceptable abbreviations for anatomical structures that are not specifically delineated in this manual, such as for specific nerves, spinal segments, ligaments, and muscles (i.e., flexor carpi ulnaris [FCU]). Also, this manual cannot possibly include all of the diagnoses and specialized medical or rehabilitation tests and terms that might be specific to your particular practice area. As health care evolves, medical terms and abbreviations can become obsolete and be replaced by new terminology. Keep current by joining professional associations and reading professional books and journals. Again, always check with your facility regarding acceptable abbreviations appropriate for your work setting.

Table 4-1
Abbreviations and Symbols

Abbreviations

Abbr.	Meaning	Abbr.	Meaning	Abbr.	Meaning
Ⓐ	assistance	BE	below elbow	CPM	continuous passive motion
ā	before	BK	below knee		
AA	Alcoholics Anonymous	BKA	below knee amputation	CPR	cardiopulmonary resuscitation
AAROM	active assisted range of motion	BM	bowel movement	CPT	Current Procedural Terminology
abd	abduction	BP	blood pressure		
add	adduction	BRP	bathroom privileges	CRPS	complex regional pain syndrome
ADD	attention deficit disorder	°C	Celsius		
ADHD	attention deficit hyperactivity disorder	c̄	with	CSF	cerebrospinal fluid
		C&S	culture and sensitivity	CST	craniosacral therapist
ADLs	activities of daily living	CA	carcinoma; cancer	CT	computed tomography
ad lib.	as desired	CABG	coronary artery bypass graft	CTD	cumulative trauma disorder
AE	above elbow	CAD	coronary artery disease		
AFO	ankle-foot orthosis	CAT	computerized axial tomography	CTR	carpal tunnel release
AIDS	acquired immunodeficiency syndrome			CTRS	Certified Therapeutic Recreation Specialist
AK	above knee	CBC	complete blood count	CTS	carpal tunnel syndrome
AKA	above knee amputation	CCU	coronary (cardiac) care unit	CVA	cerebrovascular accident
ALS	amyotrophic lateral sclerosis	CGA	contact guard assist	CXR	chest x-ray
		CHF	congestive heart failure	d	day
am, AM	morning	CHI	closed head injury	Ⓓ	dependent
AMA	against medical advice; American Medical Association	CHT	Certified Hand Therapist	D&C	dilation and curettage
		cm	centimeter	DD	developmental disability
		CMC	carpometacarpal	DIP	distal interphalangeal joint
AMB	ambulation	CNS	central nervous system		
amt.	amount	CO₂	carbon dioxide	DJD	degenerative joint disease
ant	anterior	C/O	complains of	DME	durable medical equipment
AP	anterior-posterior	cont.	continued; continue		
appt.	appointment	COPD	chronic obstructive pulmonary disease	DNR	do not resuscitate
AROM	active range of motion			D.O.	Doctor of Osteopathic Medicine
ASAP	as soon as possible	COPM	Canadian Occupational Performance Measure		
ASHD	arteriosclerotic heart disease			DOA	date of admission; dead on arrival
		COTA	Certified Occupational Therapy Assistant	DOB	date of birth
ATNR	asymmetrical tonic neck reflex			DOE	dyspnea on exertion
		CP	cerebral palsy	DPT	Doctor of Physical Therapy
Ⓑ	bilateral	CPAP	continuous positive airway pressure		
BADLs	basic activities of daily living			Dr.	doctor

(continued)

Table 4-1 (continued)
Abbreviations and Symbols

Abbreviations					
DRG	diagnostic related group	GI	gastrointestinal	lb.	pound
DRUJ	distal radioulnar joint	gm	gram	LD	learning disability; learning disorder
DTR	deep tendon reflex	GSW	gunshot wound		
DVT	deep vein thrombosis	GYN	gynecology	LE	lower extremity
Dx	diagnosis	hr.	hour	LLQ	left lower quadrant
ECG	electrocardiogram	HA, H/A	headache	LOC	loss of consciousness; level of consciousness
ECHO	echocardiogram	H&P	history and physical		
ECT	electroconvulsive therapy	HBV	hepatitis B virus	LPN	Licensed Practical Nurse
EEG	electroencephalogram	HEENT	head, eyes, ears, nose, throat	LRTI	ligament reconstruction tendinous interposition
EHR	electronic health record				
EKG	electrocardiogram	HEP	home exercise program	LTG	long-term goal
EMG	electromyogram	HHA	home health agency	LUQ	left upper quadrant
ENT	ear, nose, throat	HIPAA	Health Insurance Portability and Accountability Act	m	murmur; meter; male
EOB	edge of bed, explanation of benefits			max	maximum
				MCP, MP	metacarpophalangeal
ER	external rotation; emergency room	HIV	human immunodeficiency virus	MD	muscular dystrophy; medical doctor
e-stim	electrical stimulation	HOB	head of bed	MDS	Minimum Data Set
etc.	etcetera	HOH	hand-over-hand; hard of hearing	meds.	medications
ETOH	ethyl alcohol			MET	basal metabolic equivalent
eval.	evaluation	HP	hot pack		
exam	examination	hr.	hour	mg	milligram
ext.	extension	HR	heart rate	MHz	megahertz
°F	Fahrenheit	HRT	hormone replacement therapy	MI	myocardial infarction
F	Fair (muscle strength grade of 3)			min	minutes; minimum
		HS	bedtime	ml	milliliter
f	female	Ht	height	mm	millimeter
FBS	fasting blood sugar	HTN	hypertension	MMT	manual muscle test
FCE	functional capacity evaluation	HVPC	high volt pulsed current	mo.	month
		Hx	history	mod	moderate
FERPA	Family Educational Rights and Privacy Act	Ⓘ	independent	MRI	magnetic resonance imaging
		I&O	intake and output		
FIM™	Functional Independence Measure	IADLs	instrumental activities of daily living	MS	multiple sclerosis
				MSW	Master of Social Work
flex.	flexion	ICU	intensive care unit	MVA	motor vehicle accident
fl oz	fluid ounce	i.e.	that is	N	Normal (muscle strength grade of 5)
FM	fine motor	IEP	Individualized Education Program		
ft.	foot, feet (the measurement, not the body part)			NA	not applicable; not available
		IM	intramuscular		
F/U	follow-up	in.	inches	N/A	not applicable
FUO	fever of unknown origin	int.	internal	NAD	no acute distress
FWB	full weightbearing	IP	inpatient, interphalangeal	NBQC	narrow base quad cane
Fx	fracture	IR	internal rotation	NDT	neurodevelopmental treatment
G	Good (muscle strength grade of 4)	IV	intravenous		
		KAFO	knee-ankle-foot orthosis	neg.	negative
		kg	kilogram	NG	nasogastric
GAD	generalized anxiety disorder	Ⓛ	left	NICU	neonatal intensive care unit

(continued)

Table 4-1 (continued)
Abbreviations and Symbols

Abbreviations

NKA	no known allergy	per	by	R/O	rule out
NKDA	no known drug allergy	peri.	perineal	ROM	range of motion
NMES	neuromuscular electrical stimulation	PET	positron emission tomography	ROS	review of symptoms
NOS	not otherwise specified	PHR	personal health record	RTC	return to clinic
NPO	nothing by mouth	PIP	proximal interphalangeal	RTO	return to office
NS	no show; not seen	pm, PM	afternoon	RUGS	Resource Utilization Groups
NSAID	non-steroidal anti-inflammatory drug	PMH	past medical history	RUQ	right upper quadrant
NSR	normal sinus rhythm	PNF	proprioceptive neuro-muscular facilitation	RSD	reflex sympathetic dystrophy
NWB	non-weightbearing	PNI	peripheral nerve injury	Rx	prescription
O	objective; oriented	PNS	peripheral nervous system	$\textcircled{S}$	supervision
O_2	oxygen			$\bar{s}$	without
OA	osteoarthritis	POC	plan of care	S	subjective
OASIS	Outcome Assessment Information Set	POMR	problem-oriented medical record	SBA	stand-by assistance
				SCI	spinal cord injury
OB	obstetrics	pos.	positive	SH	social history
OBS	organic brain syndrome	post op	postoperative	SI	sensory integration
OCD	obsessive compulsive disorder	PPS	Prospective Payment System	SIDS	sudden infant death syndrome
OOB	out of bed	PRE	progressive resistive exercise	Sig:	instruction to patient
OP	outpatient			SLE	systemic lupus erythematosus
OR	operating room	pre op	preoperative		
ORIF	open reduction, internal fixation	PRN	as needed	SLP	speech-language pathologist
		pro	pronation		
OT	occupational therapist; occupational therapy	PROM	passive range of motion	SOC	start of care
		pt.	patient	SOAP	subjective, objective, assessment, plan
OTA	occupational therapy assistant	PT	physical therapist; physical therapy		
				SOB	shortness of breath
OTAS	occupational therapy assistant student	P/T	part time	SNF	skilled nursing facility
		PTA	physical therapist assis-tant, prior to admission	S/P	status post
OTC	over the counter			SSN	Social Security number
OTD	Doctor of Occupational Therapy	PTSD	post-traumatic stress disorder	STAT	immediately
				STD	sexually transmitted disease
OTR	Registered Occupational Therapist	PWB	partial weightbearing		
		qt.	quart	STG	short-term goal
OX4	oriented to time, place, person, situation	$\textcircled{R}$	right	STM	short-term memory
		R	respiration	suppos	suppository
oz	ounce	RA	rheumatoid arthritis	sup	supination
$\bar{p}$	after	RBC	red blood cell count	T	temperature; Trace (mus-cle strength grade of 1)
P	plan; posterior; pulse; Poor (muscle strength grade of 2)	re:	regarding		
		rehab	rehabilitation	TAM	total active motion
PA	posterior-anterior; physician's assistant	reps	repetitions	TB	tuberculosis
		resp	respiratory; respiration	TBI	traumatic brain injury
PAM	physical agent modality	RICE	rest, ice, compression, elevation	TEDS	thromboembolic disease stockings
PDD	pervasive developmental disorder	RLQ	right lower quadrant	TENS	transcutaneous electrical nerve stimulation
PE	physical examination	RN	Registered Nurse		

(continued)

Table 4-1 (continued)
Abbreviations and Symbols

Abbreviations

TFCC	triangular fibrocartilage complex	UA	urinalysis	WBAT	weightbearing as tolerated
ther ex	therapeutic exercise	UE	upper extremity	WBQC	wide base quad cane
THR	total hip replacement	UMN	upper motor neuron	WBC	white blood cell; white blood count
TIA	transient ischemic attack	URI	upper respiratory infection		
TKR	total knee replacement	US	ultrasound	w/c	wheelchair
TM(J)	temporomandibular (joint)	UTI	urinary tract infection	WDWN	well developed; well nourished
		VC	vital capacity		
t.o.	telephone order	VD	venereal disease	wk	week
TOS	thoracic outlet syndrome	v.o.	verbal orders	WFL	within functional limits
TPM	total passive motion	vol.	volume	WNL	within normal limits
TPR	temperature, pulse, and respiration	VS	vital signs	wt	weight
		W	watt	x or X	times
TTWB	toe-touch weightbearing	W/cm²	watt per centimeter squared	y.o.	year old
tx	treatment; traction			yr	year

Symbols

1°	primary	↓	down; downward; decrease	–	minus; negative (also abbreviated neg.)
2°	secondary; secondary to	↑	up; upward; increase		
Δ	change	↔	to and from	#	number (#1); pounds
x1, x2	of 1 person; of 2 people *Example*: "transferred to toilet c̄ min Ⓐ x2"	→	to; progressing forward; approaching	%	percent
		~	approximately	&	and
				°	degree
♀	female	@	at	"	inches
♂	male	=	equals	'	feet
>	greater than	+	plus; positive (also abbreviated pos.)	/	per
<	less than				

Worksheet 4-1
Using Abbreviations

Translate each sentence written with abbreviations into full English phrases or sentences.

1.   Pt. Ⓘ BADLs.

2.   Client reports ↓ pain Ⓡ shoulder p̄ HP.

3.   Resident w/c ↔ EOB with SBA.

4.   Client c/o pain in Ⓡ index MCP joint p̄ ~5 min PROM.

5.   Client w/c → mat c̄ sliding board max Ⓐ x2.

6.   Pt. O x 4.

7.   Client has SOB c̄ PRE.

8.   Pt. has ↓ STM and OCD, which limit IADLs.

9.   Pt. min Ⓐ AMB bed → toilet 2° ↓ balance.

10. Child's FM WFL to don AFO.

Worksheet 4-2
Using Abbreviations—Additional Practice

Shorten these notes using only the standard abbreviations in this chapter.

1. Client requires minimal assistance to stand and pull up clothing with partial weightbearing status of right lower extremity.

2. Patient is able to feed herself independently with the use of built-up utensils.

3. Client has intact sensation in both upper extremities but complains of minimal pain.

4. Client has 55 degrees of passive range of motion in the left index distal interphalangeal joint, which is within functional limits.

5. While sitting on edge of bed, client is able to put on her socks with stand-by assistance but requires moderate assistance with putting on and taking off left shoe.

6. Student is independent in wheelchair mobility and basic activities of daily living.

7. Patient requires moderate assistance of two people to transfer from wheelchair to toilet and from toilet to wheelchair.

8. Patient's toe-touch weightbearing status limits her performance of instrumental activities of daily living.

Morreale, M. J., & Borcherding, S. (2013). *The OTA's guide to documentation: Writing SOAP notes (3rd ed.)*. Thorofare, NJ: SLACK Incorporated.

Worksheet 4-3
Deciphering Doctors' Orders and Abbreviations

Translate the following abbreviations into full English phrases or sentences.

1. Dx s/p Ⓡ TKR 2° OA, WBAT
    OT 2x/wk for BADLs, IADLs

2. X-ray + Ⓛ index finger MCP Fx 2° GSW

3. 5 y.o. child has pain 2° bone CA Ⓛ LE

4. Dx Ⓡ DRUJ Fx c̄ ORIF
    OT 3x/wk for PAMs PRN, P/AROM, ADLs, CPM

5. 1° Dx PTSD, 2° Dx OCD

6. 1° Dx DJD Ⓡ hip, 2° Dx COPD & CHF

7. Dx CAD, TIA

Morreale, M. J., & Borcherding, S. (2013). *The OTA's guide to documentation: Writing SOAP notes (3rd ed.).* Thorofare, NJ: SLACK Incorporated.

Worksheet 4-4
Deciphering Doctors' Orders and Abbreviations—More Practice

Translate the following abbreviations into full English phrases or sentences.

1. Dx: PDD-NOS, ADHD
    OT: ADLs, SI, FM
    2 x/wk X 12 wk

2. EMG – Ⓡ CTS and - TOS

3. Dx: s/p Ⓛ THR, pt. NWB Ⓛ LE, OOB c̄ walker
    OT eval. and tx; ADLs, Ⓑ UE PREs
    3x/wk X 4 wks

4. MRI + TBI, VS stable, BRP

5. CXR – TB but + URI, pt. has DOE and FUO

6. Dx PTSD, MS, HBV

Morreale, M. J., & Borcherding, S. (2013). *The OTA's guide to documentation: Writing SOAP notes (3rd ed.)*. Thorofare, NJ: SLACK Incorporated.

Worksheet 4-5
Additional Practice

Shorten these notes using only the standard abbreviations in this chapter.

1. The patient participated in an occupational therapy session bedside for instruction in basic activities of daily living. She was able to perform bed mobility exercises with moderate assistance, but needed maximum assistance to put on her lower extremity garments and moderate assistance to put on upper extremity garments. She was able to go from a supine position to a sitting position with minimum assistance and from a sitting position to a standing position with moderate assistance.

2. The resident came to the occupational therapy clinic via wheelchair escort. The resident was observed to lean to his left. The resident needed verbal cues and minimum assistance in positioning his body in the wheelchair to maintain midline orientation and symmetrical posture. The resident transferred from his wheelchair to the toilet with moderate assistance of one person to help him keep his balance using a standing pivot transfer. He needed verbal cues and visual feedback from a mirror to maintain upright posture.

3. The patient was seen in the occupational therapy clinic for treatment of his left distal radioulnar joint fracture. Patient is now 10 weeks status post fracture. Patient also has an upper respiratory infection. He was seen for assessment of selected, relevant client factors for a total of 40 minutes. The left upper extremity shoulder flexion was a grade of 4 out of 5, shoulder extension was a grade of 4 out of 5, elbow flexion was a grade of 4 out of 5, elbow extension was a grade of 4 out of 5, wrist extension was a grade of 3 minus out of 5, wrist flexion was a grade of 3 minus out of 5, and grip strength was 8 pounds. The left upper extremity light touch is intact. The right upper extremity muscle grades and sensation are within functional limits.

Worksheet 4-6
Generating Abbreviations

Using the list of abbreviations in this chapter, list appropriate abbreviations for the following categories.

Lower extremity weightbearing status

1.

2.

3.

4.

5.

Different types of range of motion

1.

2.

3.

4.

5.

Physical agent modalities

1.

2.

3.

4.

5.

Morreale, M. J., & Borcherding, S. (2013). *The OTA's guide to documentation: Writing SOAP notes (3rd ed.)*. Thorofare, NJ: SLACK Incorporated.

Chapter 5

Avoiding Common Documentation Mistakes

Throughout your career as an OTA, you will encounter many opportunities to use your professional documentation skills. Of course, one essential responsibility of the OTA is to enter information in the health or education record. You will also be providing your clients with individualized written instructions for home exercise programs, safety techniques, adaptive equipment use, or other recommendations in collaboration with the OT. Other documentation tasks can include writing notes and memos to colleagues and staff. Additionally, you might even be involved with composing letters, reports, or marketing materials to send to insurance companies or other health care professionals.

Your written and verbal communication is a reflection of you, the occupational therapy practitioner. It also reflects on your department and the profession of occupational therapy as a whole. Think about what someone will infer about you from documentation that has numerous errors in spelling and grammar. Perhaps your colleagues or clients will question your credibility, your credentials, your competence, or even your intelligence. They may regard your work as sloppy or unprofessional and, thus, have less respect for you. A careless error in just one letter or word can change the meaning of a sentence or make it sound silly such as, *"Client requires increased time to transfer into the commode"* or *"The client reported hypersensitivity when his scar was palpitated."* On the other hand, documentation that is well written, grammatically correct, well organized, and neat demonstrates professionalism and pride in your work.

Make use of readily available resources such as a dictionary, thesaurus, computer program, or portable electronic devices to assist you with spelling and grammar as needed. Also, take the necessary time to write carefully and proofread your work. Rushing to complete documentation quickly can often result in substandard work and inaccuracies in copying or recording information. This could possibly lead to serious consequences for you or the client. The following sections and worksheets will help you learn to avoid some common documentation mistakes.

Morreale MJ, Borcherding S.
The OTA's Guide to Documentation:
Writing SOAP Notes, Third Edition (pp 43-52).
© 2013 SLACK Incorporated.

Quotes and Paraphrasing

There are several ways to document what your client or another person has said. It is important to objectively and accurately convey that person's intent as it relates to the client's situation. Do not embellish the information or guess at what the person might be thinking or feeling. You can quote or state what the person said exactly word for word, or you can paraphrase or summarize it. When quoting someone exactly, the person's specific words are used between a set of quotation marks. Remember that the punctuation to end the sentence stays within the quotation marks. If you are referring to the client's statement in the first person (I), the use of the letter "I" should be within the quotation marks. For example, to use a first person quote, you might write:

The client stated, "I will never be able to go back to work."

Use clinical reasoning to determine the extent of a quotation for a particular client. Consider what is clear and meaningful to enter into the health record.

The client stated, "I will never be able to go back to work. My job is very stressful."

If you, the OTA, are referring to the client in the third person (he, she), that pronoun will be outside of the quotation marks and you will just quote the exact words said. For example:

The client stated that he "will never be able to go back to work."

You can also use a combination of quotes and paraphrasing to effectively summarize and document the client's communication.

The client stated that he "will never be able to go back to work" because he considers his job too stressful.

Sometimes, you might just want to quote or emphasize a significant word or phrase. For example:

The client stated that he "will never" be able to return to his job.

The client expressed that he will not be able to resume his "very stressful" job.

If you are just paraphrasing or summarizing what another person said, you do not have to use quotation marks. Here are some examples of paraphrasing:

The client expressed doubts about returning to work.

The client stated he was uncertain about his ability to return to work.

The client stated that his job was too stressful for him to return to work.

Also, remember that an indirect question does not require a question mark.

The client asked if he would ever be able to return to work.

The client inquired about returning to work.

The client asked about coping strategies to enable return to work.

The examples on page 45 demonstrate common documentation errors and how information can be recorded in different ways.

LEARNING ACTIVITY

Ask a partner a question about leisure interests. Document your partner's response by using a quote. Then rewrite your sentence by paraphrasing what your partner said. Which of the two statements would you choose for a "real" treatment note?

Correct:

- *Patient stated, "I didn't sleep well last night."*
- *Patient stated that he "didn't sleep well last night."*
- *Patient stated that last night he didn't sleep well.*
- *Patient stated that he slept poorly last night.*

Incorrect:

- *Patient stated, "he didn't sleep well last night."*
- *Patient stated, he "didn't sleep well last night".*
- *Patient stated, I "didn't sleep well" last night.*
- *Patient stated "he slept poorly last night."*

Correct:

- *Mary stated she has "an ache" in her right hip.*
- *Mary stated, "I have an ache in my right hip."*
- *Mary stated she has discomfort in her right hip, which she describes as an ache.*
- *Mary stated that her right hip aches.*

Incorrect:

- *Mary stated, "I have an ache in her right hip."*
- *Mary stated, I have "an ache" in my right hip.*
- *Mary stated "her right hip aches."*
- *Mary stated "she has an ache in her right hip."*

Correct:

- *The client asked, "Will I be able to walk soon?"*
- *The client inquired if she would soon be able to ambulate.*
- *The client asked if she would "be able to walk soon."*
- *The client asked when she would be able to walk again.*

Incorrect:

- *The client asked "if she would be able to walk soon."*
- *The client asked if she would "be able to walk soon?"*
- *The client asked, Will I be able to walk soon?*
- *The client asked when will I walk again?*

Worksheet 5-1
Quoting and Paraphrasing

In the following statements, determine which are correct (C) or incorrect (I). Pay close attention to punctuation.

1. ___ The child stated that she was extremely hungry.
2. ___ The child stated that "she was starving."
3. ___ The child "stated I am starving."
4. ___ The child indicated that she was "starving."
5. ___ The child stated "I am starving".
6. ___ The patient asked how to put her splint on?
7. ___ The patient asked "How do I put my splint on"?
8. ___ The patient asked about the proper way to put on her splint.
9. ___ The patient asked, "How do I put my splint on?"
10. ___ The patient asked "how to put her splint on."
11. ___ The client requested a new buttonhook.
12. ___ The client asked if "she could have a new buttonhook."
13. ___ The client asked, "Can I have a new buttonhook"?
14. ___ The client asked for a new buttonhook.
15. ___ The client asked, "Can I have a new buttonhook?"
16. ___ The client stated "he felt dizzy" as he stood at the kitchen counter.
17. ___ The client reported feeling "dizzy" while standing at the kitchen counter.
18. ___ While standing at the kitchen counter, the client stated "he felt dizzy."
19. ___ The client, while standing at the kitchen counter, stated I feel "dizzy."
20. ___ The client reported dizziness while standing at the kitchen counter.

Mini Worksheet 5-2
Spelling

Students frequently misspell some common words used in occupational therapy documentation. For each of the pairs below, place a check mark next to the word that is spelled correctly.

1. ___ defered   ___ deferred   7. ___ recieve   ___ receive
2. ___ definately   ___ definitely   8. ___ pnumonia   ___ pneumonia
3 ___ dining   ___ dinning   9. ___ rotator cup   ___ rotator cuff
4. ___ excercise   ___ exercise   10. ___ tolorate   ___ tolerate
5. ___ parrafin   ___ paraffin   11 ___ therapy puddy ___ therapy putty
6. ___ transfering   ___ transferring   12 ___ independent   ___ independant

Worksheet 5-3
Spelling—More Practice

Place a check mark next to the word that is spelled correctly.

1. ___ counseling   ___ counselling
2. ___ diarrhea   ___ diarrea
3. ___ hemhorrage   ___ hemorrhage
4. ___ benefit   ___ benifit
5. ___ interfered   ___ interferred
6. ___ eyesite   ___ eyesight
7. ___ pullies   ___ pulleys
8. ___ extention   ___ extension
9. ___ hygeine   ___ hygiene
10. ___ preparation   ___ preperation
11. ___ therapeutic   ___ theraputic
12. ___ flexability   ___ flexibility
13. ___ strength   ___ strenth
14. ___ assymetrical   ___ asymmetrical
15. ___ toilet   ___ toliet
16. ___ leisure   ___ liesure
17. ___ nauseous   ___ nauseus

Morreale, M. J., & Borcherding, S. (2013). *The OTA's guide to documentation: Writing SOAP notes (3rd ed.).* Thorofare, NJ: SLACK Incorporated.

Worksheet 5-4
Using Words Correctly

Students often misuse certain words that sound similar. Complete the following sentences by choosing the correct word from the two choices provided in parentheses.

1. The home health _____ gave the patient a shower. (aid or aide)

2. The client refused to _____ the doctor's diagnosis. (accept or except)

3. The traumatic brain injury will have a tremendous _____ on activities of daily living. (affect or effect)

4. If the client falls, she probably will _____ her hip due to osteoporosis. (brake or break)

5. The patient became short of _____ after ambulating to the bathroom. (breath or breathe)

6. The client stated she wanted to _____ ten pounds. (lose or loose)

7. The patient injured her _____ right hand, which prevented her from writing. (dominant or dominate)

8. The occupational therapy room is _____ down the hallway than the physical therapy room. (farther or further)

9. The _____ caseload consists of 10 clients, as compared to 15 clients last week. (currant or current)

10. The OTR asked the patient to _____ the scissors down on the table. (lay or lie)

11. The weight of the pan was more _____ the patient could manage. (than or then)

12. The clients in the craft group put _____ projects away in the closet. (their or there)

13. The child was able to remain quiet and _____ while standing in line. (stationary or stationery)

14. The _____ of the school attended the IEP meeting. (principal or principle)

Morreale, M. J., & Borcherding, S. (2013). *The OTA's guide to documentation: Writing SOAP notes (3rd ed.).* Thorofare, NJ: SLACK Incorporated.

Worksheet 5-5
Using Words Correctly—More Practice

Choose the correct word from the two choices provided in parentheses.

1. The client has difficulty _____ the steering wheel. (griping or gripping)

2. The client was able to navigate his wheelchair throughout the store's _____ without knocking anything over. (isles or aisles)

3. The patient refused to take _____ responsibility for his actions. (personal or personnel)

4. The patient reported pain when his biceps muscle was _____ by the OTA. (palpitated or palpated)

5. The client was able to _____ all bathing tasks without assistance. (perform or preform)

6. The child asked for a _____ of candy. (peace or piece)

7. The client had difficulty swallowing liquids due to _____ . (dysphagia or dysphasia)

8. The student was denied _____ to the client's medical record. (excess or access)

9. The client followed the OTA's _____ and purchased a shower chair. (advice or advise)

10. A buttonhook can be a useful assistive _____ for clients with impaired dexterity. (device or devise)

11. The student was _____ at playing the violin. (adapt or adept)

12. The client developed a lung infection due to _____ of food. (aspiration or inspiration)

13. The resident was very _____ during transfers as she would not wait for the wheelchair to be properly positioned and locked before trying to stand up. (compulsive or impulsive)

Capitals

When in doubt regarding the use of capitals, always refer to a medical or college dictionary. Some of the more commonly confused situations regarding capitals are listed below and, according to the *Merriam-Webster's Guide to Punctuation and Style* (Merriam-Webster, 2001), the following rules pertain:

Capitalized	Example	Not Capitalized	Example
Proper names in medical terminology	Parkinson disease, Babinski sign, Heimlich maneuver	Common nouns in medical terminology	measles, virus, flu, hysterectomy, biceps
Trade names of products and medications	Pampers diapers, Jobst glove, Advil	Generic drugs and products	disposable diapers, compression glove, aspirin
Specific organizations	American Occupational Therapy Association	Generic organizations	study group, a book club, craft group
Academic degrees and professional designations after the person's name	Marie Morreale, OTR/L, CHT	General degrees or generic professional designations	an associate's degree, an occupational therapist
Exact test titles	Canadian Occupational Performance Measure	Generic tests	range of motion assessment, a cognitive evaluation, a short-term memory test
Specific department proper names	Healthy Hospital Occupational Therapy Department	Generic department names	an occupational therapy department, rehab department
Official titles as part of a name	Dr. Jones, Reverend Smith	Generic or descriptive titles	the doctor's office, the clergyman

Mini Worksheet 5-6
Capitals

Underline the words that do not correctly follow the rules for capitals.

1.   The OTA put the chart on the Occupational Therapist's desk.

2.   The Patient was going to see his Doctor this afternoon.

3.   The OT Aide used velcro and Scotch Tape to fix Mrs. Smith's lapboard during the occupational therapy session.

4.   The Doctor spoke to the child who has Chicken Pox.

5.   The OTA Student performed a Sensory Test on the client.

6.   The client took Tylenol and Antacids before his Business Meeting.

7.   The Nurse told the new mother that the infant has down syndrome.

8.   The Physical Therapist informed the OTA that their client was admitted to the Hospital due to Pneumonia.

9.   The Occupational therapy assistant worked in the outpatient department.

10. The OT used the Miller assessment for preschoolers to assess the child with Autism.

Morreale, M. J., & Borcherding, S. (2013). *The OTA's guide to documentation: Writing SOAP notes (3rd ed.).* Thorofare, NJ: SLACK Incorporated.

Verb Tenses

Choose and use one verb tense within a paragraph. Consider the following:

> The OTA **has helped** Joe's fine motor skills; the PT **helped** Joe's balance. The special educator **had worked** with Joe so he could learn the school routine. The classroom aide **works** very closely with him every day.

The above paragraph uses four different verb tenses: present perfect, past, past perfect, and present. Instead, it is better to choose and use only one verb tense.

Pronouns

Be careful to make the pronoun reference clear. If you say, *"Jane and Mary agree that her skills are improving,"* it is not clear if the "her" refers to Jane or refers to Mary. It is better to say, *"Jane and Mary agree that Mary's skills are improving."* Another incorrect example is *"The OT's student put his goniometer in his lab coat pocket,"* as it is not clear whose goniometer or whose pocket is being referred to. It would be better to say, *"The OT student put the OT's goniometer in the OT's lab coat pocket."*

Another common student error is using pronouns that don't agree with the subject to which they refer. For example, it is incorrect to write, *"One person in the group wasn't able to complete their craft project."* Instead, it should read, *"One person in the group wasn't able to complete his craft project"* (or *"her craft project"* if referring to a female).

You must also determine if the subject and pronoun are singular or plural for consistency. Consider this incorrect statement, *"They will hurt themself if they lift too much weight."* The correct version is *"They will hurt themselves if they lift too much weight."*

Plurals and Possessives

The proper way to indicate plurals or possessives can sometimes seem confusing. We will now look at several situations that are commonly prone to errors. According to the *Publication Manual of the American Psychological Association* (American Psychological Association [APA], 2010), to indicate the plural of an abbreviation, usually just the letter "s" is added. For example:

- *The OTs each supervised two OTAs.*
- *The MDs wanted to use the conference room.*
- *The three OTAs all graduated from the same college.*
- *The OTA presented an in-service on body mechanics to the four RNs.*

Remember that when you are showing that something belongs to one person or object (singular possessive), most of the time you use an apostrophe before the letter "s." Here are some examples:

- *The client's right hand was minimally edematous.*
- *That chair's armrests are broken.*
- *The OTA's goniometer is in her desk.*
- *The patient's commode was placed next to his bed.*

When you have more than one person or object and want to indicate that something belongs to all of them (plural possessive), the apostrophe goes after the letter "s." For example:

- *The clients' charts were in the file cabinet.*
- *The OTA students' lunches were free in the hospital cafeteria.*
- *The occupational therapy assistants' treatment notes were cosigned by their supervisors.*
- *The OTAs' patients were all in the waiting room.*
- *Three of the patients' lunch trays were missing utensils.*

Mini Worksheet 5-7
Pronouns, Plurals, Possessives

Look at the following sentences and determine the incorrect components in each sentence.

1. The three client's appointments were all canceled today because their OTA was ill.

2. The OTAs lab coat was new.

3. The OTA students resumé was reviewed by the OT.

4. The childs parent's attended the therapy session.

5. The children almost hurt theirselves when they collided with each other in the hallway.

6. The nurses patient gave them all flowers.

7. The PT's and OT's had the day off.

8. The occupational therapists' paperwork was on her desk.

9. One of the client's lost their splint.

10. The OT took the OTAs lab coat home by mistake.

11. Sarah told her teacher's she did the homework by themselves.

12. The broken wheelchairs were repaired by the two PTA's.

Now you are ready to begin writing SOAP notes. Always remember that your documentation is a reflection of you as both an individual and occupational therapy professional. Make a concerted effort to use correct spelling, punctuation, and grammar in all of your professional writing. When in doubt, refer to a dictionary, spellchecker, or style manual to assure accuracy. The rest of this manual will take you step-by-step through the process of writing SOAP notes and help you to develop clinical reasoning skills. You will be soon be thinking and writing like an OTA.

Morreale, M. J., & Borcherding, S. (2013). *The OTA's guide to documentation: Writing SOAP notes (3rd ed.)*. Thorofare, NJ: SLACK Incorporated.

Chapter 6

Writing the "S"—Subjective

The first section of the SOAP note contains **SUBJECTIVE** information obtained from the client. This "S" section expresses the client's perspective regarding his or her condition or treatment. Subjective data is information that cannot necessarily be verified or measured during the intervention session. In this section, the occupational therapy practitioner records the client's report of limitations, concerns and problems, as well as what the client communicated that was relevant to treatment. This can include statements regarding significant complaints of pain; fatigue; or expressions of feelings, attitudes, concerns, goals, and plans. Appropriate, direct quotes are often used in the subjective section of the SOAP note. In this case, it is understood that the statement comes from the individual receiving the therapy, unless otherwise stated. This subjective information will have more significance and relevance to the rest of your note if it specifically pinpoints an issue rather than just noting a vague or general comment from the client. For instance, if the client tells you, "My hand hurts," you may probe further, asking, "Where does it hurt?" or "When does it hurt?" or "Describe what it feels like." This will allow your note to communicate more detailed information on the individual's condition by recording the client's own description or perception: *"Client states he has sharp pain in his Ⓡ thumb and index MP joints when he uses a hammer or wrench."* You may quote, paraphrase, or summarize what the client said. Review Chapter 5 for detailed information regarding the use of proper grammar and punctuation for direct and indirect quotes.

Examples of "S" Statements

- *"I don't need therapy."*
- *Student stated she has difficulty changing in and out of her gym clothes within the allotted time in class.*
- *Client reports "pins and needles" in Ⓡ hand when driving >15 minutes.*
- *Client reports feeling frustrated because her short arm cast interferes with ability to perform home management tasks.*
- *Patient expressed doubts about ever getting better and then began to cry.*
- *Client reports, "I keep losing my patience at home and yelling at my family, and I don't know what to do about it."*
- *"I can't tie my shoes or zip my coat because my thumb is too stiff."*
- *Veteran reports that he has frequent flashbacks of combat duty that wake him up at night.*
- *Child reports that she is too embarrassed to wear her leg brace and splints because the other students make fun of her.*

Morreale MJ, Borcherding S.
*The OTA's Guide to Documentation:
Writing SOAP Notes, Third Edition (pp 53-57).*
© 2013 SLACK Incorporated.

- *Patient expresses a desire to return to her factory job as soon as possible. She is also concerned about the financial implications of her inability to work 2° her injury.*
- *Client reports being fearful of leaving her family and moving to a group home.*
- *Client reports that his doctor has ordered "some home care for a few days to work on transfers."*
- *Client reported that she has been performing her shoulder exercises twice daily without any discomfort. She also stated that she can now reach items in her upper kitchen cabinets with her Ⓡ UE.*
- *Client called the emergency line last night to report a burning sensation in her "gut," which made her afraid she was going to die. Today she reports that she has been worrying about dying and has not showered since the day before yesterday.*
- *Resident expressed that she has experienced several episodes of bladder incontinence and, therefore, does not like leaving her room.*
- *Client stated, "I feel so stressed out about losing my job that I can't concentrate or sleep. I don't feel like myself anymore." She also reported that gardening and volunteer work are her primary coping strategies, and that she would like to learn more about relaxation techniques.*
- *Student stated that her hand gets very tired when she writes.*
- *Client reports that stress and anxiety about losing his job is the reason he drinks alcohol excessively.*

Sometimes the client is not able to speak or does not make any relevant comments. In such cases, include that information in the "S" section. For example:

- *Client unable to communicate due to aphasia.*
- *Client did not speak without cueing.*
- *Patient communicated using his message board that he wants to be able to walk again.*
- *Resident does not clearly verbalize during treatment, but smiles and nods appropriately when asked questions.*

In certain instances, the "S" part of the SOAP note might reflect an important statement, problem, or concern that the client's caregiver or family communicates to the OTA regarding the client. Also, when treating infants and very young children, you may report what the parent or guardian says. For example:

- *Mother reports child will only tolerate mashed or pureed foods due to his oral sensitivity.*
- *Caregiver reports client refuses to wear her splint.*
- *Although client denies taking alcohol and drugs, her husband states, "I am really concerned that she is eventually going to kill herself. She will not stop drinking and taking cocaine."*
- *Parent reported child has an ear infection and is "very cranky today." She also expressed concern that the child's recurrent ear infections may necessitate surgery.*
- *Daughter reports client lives with her and sometimes forgets to turn off the stove. Daughter states she works full-time and is concerned that her mother is home alone during the day and could hurt herself or start a fire.*

The "S" section is usually reserved for the client's point of view except for situations with infants, people who are unable to communicate, and special circumstances. If a client is deaf or only speaks a different language, it is important to have someone present who can interpret or translate all communication between the client and occupational therapy practitioner. This should also be recorded in the note.

Common Errors

Not Using Communication Time With the Client Effectively

A common error that new OTAs make in gathering subjective information is in failing to make good use of communication with the client during intervention sessions. It is certainly important to make the client feel comfortable and at ease. However, rather than using most of the therapy time to talk socially, a good OTA will use the time to listen effectively and to ask questions that will elicit pertinent information about the client's attitudes and concerns. This information can then be used to ensure effective treatment as well as appropriate documentation. Instead of discussing the weather or a professional sporting event, why not ask your client how he thinks he is doing in therapy or what his feelings are related to his upcoming discharge placement? As OTAs gain experience, they begin to use the intervention session to obtain relevant data regarding such things as occupational history, functional status, prior level of functioning, priorities, motivation, and family support. Effective communication during treatment can seem just like a conversation on the surface. But, as a skilled OTA, you are carefully directing the conversation to topics that are meaningful to client care rather than allowing it to remain superficial. Use this opportunity to expand the client's occupational profile and gather information that is vital to providing the very best occupational therapy possible. When conversing with your client, guide the discussion to your client's history, problems, needs, concerns, strengths, support systems, living situation, and goals for treatment. Without knowing these things from your client's point of view, you will have difficulty planning effective interventions. When an OTA does not listen effectively during treatment, the "S" may read:

- *Client talked about grandchildren visiting.*
- *Resident reported she was wearing a new dress today.*
- *Pt. stated that his lunch tasted very good.*

While these statements are within the scope of the "S," they are not particularly helpful pieces of information to spend time and space reporting.

Not Writing Concise, Coherent Statements

Another common error new OTAs make when writing the subjective section of the note is that of simply listing any remarks the client makes about his condition.

For example, during one treatment session, the client said the following:

- *"I'm wobbly as can be today."*
- *"I can't feel anything with my hands."*
- *Client expressed dizziness after bending down to touch the floor while in a seated position.*
- *Client acknowledged improvement in his sitting balance in comparison to the previous week.*

These statements generally involve stability, balance, and safety issues. While the quotations are a very objective way of reporting information and all of the remarks are relevant to the intervention session, it is more effective to summarize the client's statements more concisely and coherently. Rather than listing each of these statements separately in the "S" section of the note, organize and record them in a more professional manner. For example:

- *Client reported lack of sensation in both hands and dizziness in sitting position with dynamic movement (a "wobbly" sensation). He also acknowledged improvement in sitting balance since last week.*
- *Client acknowledged improved sitting balance compared to previous week. However, he expressed dizziness after bending down while sitting, and reported feeling "wobbly." Client also reported inability to feel anything with his hands.*

In the next two exercises, you will have the opportunity to select coherent and concise "S" statements.

Worksheet 6-1
Choosing a Subjective Statement

A female client is recovering after a Ⓛ CVA. This observation note was written after one of her occupational therapy intervention sessions.

O: *Client participated in 45-minute OT session in hospital room to ↑ AROM in Ⓡ shoulder, activity tolerance, UE strength, and dynamic standing balance, in order to ↑ independence in ADL tasks.*

   BADL: *Client was instructed on safety techniques and adaptive equipment use for toileting. Client required use of bilateral grab bars in bathroom to sit ↔ stand safely. Client first attempted to stand while pulling on walker and one grab bar. Client was instructed on safety issues and the use of bilateral grab bars, which she reported understanding.*

   Performance Skills: *Client sit → stand CGA for balance. Client worked on activity tolerance, dynamic standing balance, and ↑ AROM in Ⓡ shoulder by hanging items in closet for 5 minutes before needing to sit and rest 2 minutes. She then participated in activities to ↑ dynamic standing balance by donning a bathrobe while standing CGA for balance. After a 1-minute rest, client continued activities to ↑ dynamic standing balance and safety in ADL activities by pushing wheeled walker while picking up objects from floor c̄ a reacher.*

   Client Factors: *AROM right shoulder abduction <90°. PROM Ⓡ shoulder abduction WNL.*

The treatment session included all of the following. Which would be best to use as the subjective section of the SOAP note?

1. *Client remarked that her grandson will be coming to visit later in the week, and that she will be very glad to see him.*

2. *Client was cooperative and engaged in social conversation throughout the treatment session.*

3. *Client reports that she feels "pretty good" today.*

4. *Client says she has difficulty moving Ⓡ UE, although she does not know why it will not move. She reports, "It really doesn't hurt. It's just tight."*

5. *Nursing staff report client is unsafe to toilet self independently.*

Morreale, M. J., & Borcherding, S. (2013). *The OTA's guide to documentation: Writing SOAP notes (3rd ed.).* Thorofare, NJ: SLACK Incorporated.

Worksheet 6-2
Writing Concise, Coherent Statements

Your client is recovering from a Ⓛ total hip replacement. During an occupational therapy intervention session, the client makes the following statements.

- *"I used that dressing stick and sock aid like you showed me to get dressed without bending down this morning."*

- *"It's getting easier for me to get dressed now."*

- *"My hip doesn't hurt when I stand up or sit down, especially with that new toilet seat you got for me."*

- *"My daughter said they delivered all that bathroom equipment to her house yesterday."*

Using these statements, write your own concise and organized version for the "S" portion of the SOAP note.

S:

Morreale, M. J., & Borcherding, S. (2013). *The OTA's guide to documentation: Writing SOAP notes (3rd ed.)*. Thorofare, NJ: SLACK Incorporated.

Chapter 7

Writing the "O"—Objective

The second part of the note is the **OBJECTIVE** section. This is where you will record all measurable, quantifiable, and observable data obtained during your client's occupational therapy session. In this section, your note presents a mental picture or synopsis of the entire encounter. Once you begin looking at things with your professional eyes, they can look and seem quite different. Instead of simply seeing a child playing with a toy, you now begin to make skilled observations such as noting the child's asymmetrical posture, hand preference, balance, ability to cross midline, and pinch and grasp patterns. A student or novice OTA may have difficulty deciding what kind of material to include and what to omit in the "O" section. At first your "O" may tend to be longer than that of an experienced OTA, but with time you will learn to write notes that are both complete and concise.

Guidelines for Writing Good Observations

Begin With a Statement About the Setting and Purpose of the Activity

Start with the term for *"client"* that is most appropriate for your facility such as resident, infant, child, student, patient, veteran, consumer, etc. Follow that with terminology noting the client's active participation in therapy (Gateley & Borcherding, 2012; Sames, 2010). For example, Sames (2010) recommends that, instead of writing that the client was "seen" during the session, it is preferable to use the words "participated in" (Sames, 2010, p. 10). As third-party payers may balk at paying for continued therapy if it appears the client is just a passive observer, this is an important distinction (Gateley & Borcherding, 2012; Sames, 2010). You may use similar words in the opening sentence such as *"client engaged in"* or *"client worked on."* Next, indicate where the therapy took place and the purpose of the therapy session.

If your intervention activities are **occupation-based tasks**, use the following format for your opening sentence:

Client participated in ____ -minute session in _____ for _____.
                  #   (In what setting)   (Purpose of the treatment session)

For example:

- *Resident participated in 45-minute session bedside for instruction in compensatory dressing techniques.*
- *Child engaged in 30-minute OT session in classroom to improve ability to use computer keyboard in class.*
- *Client participated in 30-minute cooking group in OT kitchen for skilled instruction in compensatory techniques for meal preparation.*

Morreale MJ, Borcherding S.
The OTA's Guide to Documentation:
Writing SOAP Notes, Third Edition (pp 59-68).
© 2013 SLACK Incorporated.

Some facilities require that you document the number of minutes for the total occupational therapy session or for each specific occupational therapy service the client receives. Your recorded minutes are typically used for billing purposes, such as determining the correct CPT code or if questions arise regarding the amount or specific type of occupational therapy treatment the client received. Time notations may also be used to track the productivity of individual staff members or the entire department. Facilities that do not charge for occupational therapy by the number of minutes may not require that you document the length of time a client was seen. However, you do still need to document the skilled services that were provided.

If the session is centered on improving **client factors** such as active range of motion, strengthening, activity tolerance, or dynamic balance, then add a reference to the **relevant area of occupation** in the opening line:

Client participated in _____ -minute session in _____ to work on _____ for _____ .
    #   (In what setting)   (Purpose)   (For what expected
                                                                                                  functional gain)

For example:

- *Student engaged in 30-minute therapy session in OT room to promote development of dynamic tripod grasp for **handwriting**.*
- *Child engaged in 45-minute OT session at his home to work on increasing selective attention and fine motor manipulation as a prerequisite to **enhanced play and BADL tasks**.*
- *Client participated in 60-minute session in hospital room for skilled instruction in energy conservation for **IADLs**.*
- *Consumer participated in role-play activity for 30 minutes in assertion group in order to explore alternative ways to get his **social needs** met.*
- *Client participated in 30-minute current events group to decrease social anxiety when **interacting with peers**.*
- *Pt. participated in 60-minute OT session in clinic for application of moist heat, P/AROM, and strengthening exercises to Ⓡ UE in order to restore skills needed for **return to work**.*
- *Resident participated in ½ hour UE exercise group to ↑ strength for **w/c mobility**.*

Occupational therapy practitioners do not always write the "O" this exact way. In some instances, you might choose to switch your sentence around slightly:

- *In sensory integration playroom, child participated in OT activities for 30 minutes to address sensory defensiveness in classroom activities.*
- *In OT kitchen, client worked on standing activities for 15 minutes in order to increase activity tolerance for cooking.*
- *In order to improve interpersonal skills and promote leisure skills development, pt. participated in 30-minute OT craft group.*

Show Your Skill

It is important to show the need for your skill as an OTA in the very first sentence of your "O." As previously mentioned, instead of saying, "*Client seen for 45 minutes bedside for dressing,*" it is better to indicate active client engagement (Gateley & Borcherding, 2012; Sames, 2010) and then clearly identify the specific skilled occupational therapy services implemented. You might say:

- *Client participated in 45-minute BADL session bedside for **instruction in compensatory dressing techniques**.*
- *Client engaged in therapy 45 minutes bedside to **facilitate attention to Ⓛ side during self-care activities**.*
- *Resident participated in therapy 45 minutes bedside for **instruction in adaptive equipment use to increase safety in BADL tasks**.*

Here are some more examples showing the skill of an occupational therapy practitioner:

- *Client engaged in 30 minutes of therapy in OT kitchen to work on improving **time management**.*
- *For 30 minutes in technology clinic, child and parents participated in **assistive technology training for classroom activities**.*
- *Pt. participated in 1-hour session in OT clinic for **fabrication of Ⓛ cock-up splint to ↓ pain during ADLs**.*
- *In classroom, child participated in OT 45 minutes for **adaptation of backpack to enable Ⓘ use**.*
- *Resident participated 30 minutes in OT life skills group for **instruction in stress management techniques**.*

Follow the Opening Sentence With a Summary of What You Observed

After the setting and purpose have been established, you will discuss the intervention you have just completed, either in chronological order or organized into categories. Some notes work best when reported chronologically, and others work better with categories.

Organization of the "O"

There are different ways to organize the information gleaned from your observations. One way is to present the information chronologically and discuss each intervention or event in the order it occurred during that particular session.

> *Resident participated in 45-minute OT session bedside for skilled instruction in BADLs and to ↑ activity tolerance. Once set up, resident was able to wash face and upper body with min Ⓐ and use of a wash mitt while sitting on EOB. Client also was instructed in use of long handle hairbrush and electric toothbrush. She demonstrated ability to use these items to perform grooming tasks with min Ⓐ to open toothpaste and two 60-second rest periods. Resident then applied make-up with min Ⓐ to open containers while sitting up in bed. She expressed satisfaction regarding being finally able to participate in a "normal morning routine."*

Alternately, you may choose to organize your information into categories.

When categorizing your information, choose the categories that make the most sense for your note. For example, suppose that today you saw a home care client for a cooking session in her kitchen. She is recovering from a total hip replacement (THR) and needs to be able to prepare a light meal independently once her home health aide is discontinued. You do not know her level of safety awareness or her ability to perform all steps of the activities while using a walker. You wonder if her activity tolerance and upper extremity function are adequate for cooking, and you also want to assess her judgment, problem solving, and ability to adhere to THR precautions. You choose the following categories:

- Functional mobility
- Upper extremity AROM and strength
- Activity tolerance
- Cognition

Your note might look like this:

> **O**: *Client participated in 60-minute OT session at home for skilled instruction in compensatory cooking techniques and safety assessment.*
> ***Functional Mobility**: Client used walker to maneuver throughout kitchen and she needed min verbal cues to position walker appropriately for reaching objects in cabinets and refrigerator. Client was instructed in use of walker basket and wheeled cart to transport items.*
> ***UE AROM and Strength**: WFL for reaching items in drawers and upper cabinets and putting dishes in the sink Ⓘ. UE strength adequate for opening refrigerator door, using manual can opener, and pouring soup in and out of small pot. Client required min Ⓐ to use reacher to obtain item from bottom shelf in refrigerator.*
> ***Activity Tolerance**: Client demonstrated ability to stand Ⓘ for 10 minutes to heat soup at stove and make sandwich at counter. Client required a 5-minute break then stood at sink for 5 minutes to wash dishes.*
> ***Cognitive**: Client able to respond to verbal instructions and questions with correct response 3/3 times. Client stated she did not think it would be safe for her to use the oven at this time and would use the toaster oven instead. Client able to problem solve and safely adhere to all THR precautions.*

There is no list of "correct" categories. You must use your clinical judgment to determine what is appropriate to include, summarize, or categorize. If the client has no deficits in a particular area, it is not necessary to address that category in the note. In choosing categories, you could use the *Framework-II* categories (AOTA, 2008b) as these are useful in any practice setting.

- Areas of occupation
- Performance skills
- Performance patterns
- Client factors
- Activity demands
- Context and environment

In some instances, those *Framework-II* categories may too broad for your purposes. You might choose subcategories or other areas that relate more specifically to your client and your practice setting. You may want to consider some of the following:

- **Basic and instrumental ADL task performance**: Note how each of the performance skills and client factors observed impact completion of specific ADL tasks. Include assist levels and required set-up, adaptive equipment/durable medical equipment, positioning, compensatory techniques, and methods used. Also include extent and type of cuing and response, rest periods needed, family/caregiver education, and client's response to the intervention provided.

- **Education and work**: Note activity demands and any adaptive equipment, assistive technology, or modifications needed for school, work, or volunteer activities. Address time management, organizational skills, and ability to perform educational or job-related tasks. Consider career and transitional planning as well as the development of vocational skills.

- **Leisure and play**: Consider physical, cognitive, psychosocial and developmental factors regarding participation in leisure activities. Note barriers to play and leisure, skill development, and appropriateness of leisure time and choices.

- **Posture and balance**: Note whether balance was static or dynamic for sitting and standing. Consider whether the client leans in one direction, has rotated posture, or has even or uneven weight distribution. Notice position of the head, upper extremities, trunk, and symmetry. Note what feedback, cues, or devices were needed to maintain or restore balance.

- **Coordination and dexterity**: Note if dominant hand is affected, type of prehension patterns used, ability to grasp and maintain grasp of objects without dropping, functional reach and purposeful release, proximal control, precision handling, in-hand manipulation, gross versus fine motor ability. Consider ability to manage bimanual tasks.

- **Swelling or edema**: Describe location and type of edema and give girth or volumetric measurements if possible.

- **Pain**: Describe or quantify the pain and note the frequency and location. Consider how pain impacts the areas of occupation and performance patterns.

- **Muscle, bone, joint, and sensory functions**: Note specific type and location of sensory losses and consider whether PROM, AROM, strength, and structural alignment are adequate for performing occupational tasks.

- **Movement patterns in affected extremities**: Note motor planning, tremors, tone (i.e., rigidity, flaccidity, hypotonicity, hypertonicity, and synergy pattern). Also describe facilitation or stabilization required, atypical body movement, substitution, or compensatory motions.

- **Ability to follow instructions**: Note attention, behavior, type and amount of instruction required (such as physical, verbal or visual cuing), and ability to follow one-, two-, or three-step directions.

- **Cognition and perception**: Report on task initiation; appropriateness of verbal, written, or motor responses; approach to the task; ability to stay on task; sequencing; orientation (identifying time, place, person, and situation); requirements for cuing; number of steps successfully completed in task; judgment (recognition of impairments, impulsivity, safety); and ability to correct errors. Note if client has unilateral neglect, impaired spatial relations, or difficulty crossing midline.

- **Functional mobility**: Note the kind of assistance, cues, adapted technique, special devices, or equipment required for the client to reposition self in bed, walk, transfer, propel a wheelchair, and use public transportation or drive.

- **Activity tolerance**: Note level of energy and endurance during tasks and impact on occupational performance.

- **Psychosocial factors**: Note client's overall appearance, hygiene, affect, mood, body image, and appropriateness of behavior. Also note family or community support, coping mechanisms, intrapersonal and interpersonal skills, and ability to adapt and make realistic discharge decisions for self.

Look at the following client situation and two different examples of how the "O" part of the note might be written for this client.

Julie is a 27-year-old mother of two children ages 2 and 4. She is employed in a manufacturing job that involves lifting 30-pound boxes. She is currently unable to work due to back pain from a herniated disc in her lumbar area. She complains of pain when doing her housework and tells you that she wants to be able to perform IADLs and work tasks without pain. As part of her occupational profile, the OT delegates several tasks to the OTA that need to be observed and modified. You, the OTA, are asked to have this client demonstrate some performance skills for IADLs and work. You watch her take items from the refrigerator, wash the dishes, sweep and vacuum the floor, and lift a box from the floor to a chair. You observe that her body mechanics are poor and determine that she would benefit from client education. If you reported on your session using chronological order, you might say:

O: *Client participated in 30-minute session in OT clinic for assessment of low back pain and instruction in proper body mechanics. Client sits asymmetrically with weight shifted to her Ⓛ hip. Client demonstrated the way she usually removes items from the refrigerator, washes dishes, cleans the floors, and lifts. She was then instructed in proper body mechanics for completing those tasks (using a golfer's lift, squats, stepping toward the item she wishes to retrieve, facing the load and keeping it close to her body). Client demonstrated techniques correctly and was given education materials to remind her of correct positioning.*

If you wanted to put the same information into categories, you might say:

O: *Client participated in 30-minute session in OT clinic for assessment of low back pain and instruction in proper body mechanics.*
*   **Bending and Lifting**: Client demonstrated her usual way of moving items from low surfaces to higher ones, demonstrating incorrect body mechanics in back extension and bending at the waist. After instruction in using golfer's lift or squat, client demonstrated ability to use these techniques correctly in lifting and work activities after two attempts.*
*   **Transporting**: Client exhibited torque in the spine in transporting items such as dishes. After instruction in sidestepping, facing the load and keeping it close to the body, client demonstrated proper use of these techniques with less reported pain.*
*   **Reaching**: IADL tasks such as sweeping and vacuuming also habitually performed with rotation and over-extension of the back. After instruction and demonstration of moving the body rather than overextending the arms, and keeping the load close to the body, client demonstrated correct body mechanics in performing reaching tasks with decreased pain.*
*   **Client Education**: Client given educational material to remind her of correct positioning for task and client reported that she understood what to do.*

In this case, the chronological note works better because there is some repetition in the categorized version, and the categorized version is also longer. However, some notes are better if they are divided into sections. Categories help an inexperienced OTA to focus on the performance skills the client is demonstrating rather than the treatment media that is being used to facilitate these skills. It also helps other professionals to find pertinent information more quickly when they read your note. Complete Worksheet 7-1 to review a chronological note that would work better in categories.

Additional Guidelines for Writing Good Observations

Don't Duplicate Services

Make sure that your intervention is **specific to occupational therapy** as third-party payers will not pay for duplication of services. While there will naturally be some overlap among rehabilitation disciplines, make sure you record what occupational therapy is doing differently. For example, the physical therapist might be working with a client on ambulation with the goal of teaching the use of an ambulation device or working on ambulation distance. Occupational therapy might work with this same client using the ambulation device for a **specific functional activity**, such as loading the dishwasher safely or getting clothes out of a closet. If both occupational therapy and physical therapy are working on transfers, perhaps physical therapy is working on transfers to the mat or wheelchair and occupational therapy is working on transfers to the toilet or tub using adaptive equipment. If the speech therapist has the client reading a newspaper to facilitate articulation and language, the occupational therapy practitioner might be using the newspaper to facilitate cognitive skills and functional problem solving, such as locating classified ads or the movie schedule.

Make Your Note Professional, Concise, and Specific

The "O" section does not always need to be written in complete sentences, but it does need to make sense. Give complete information in the most concise form possible. It is imperative that certain details be included. For example, ROM must be specified as passive, active, or assistive and must indicate the action and joint at which the movement occurred. UE or LE must indicate which UE or LE. Level of physical or verbal assistance must be specified if assistance was given.

When you are documenting test results, it is helpful to put them into a chart like the following one, rather than burying them in a narrative.

Sensation in Ⓛ hand:	
Hot/cold:	Intact
Sharp/dull:	Impaired over volar surface, intact over dorsal surface
Stereognosis:	Absent

As you can see in the following examples, appropriate changes in wording can make your notes sound more professional and succinct. For more suggestions, refer to Table 7-1.

Rather than saying: *"Resident flopped down onto bed short of breath, closed her eyes, and moaned. Resident reclined in bed with min Ⓐ to position herself."*

You might say: *"Client observed to be fatigued following therapy session and required min Ⓐ for positioning in bed."*

Rather than saying: *"Veteran grabbed onto the trapeze and used it in order to sit up."*
You might say: *"Supine → sit using trapeze."*

Rather than saying: *"Client put the board in place to make a sliding board transfer."*
You might say: *"Client positioned sliding board for transfer."*

Table 7-1
Using Professional Language

Rather than saying...	You might say...	
Good arm (or leg)	Strong arm (or leg) Unaffected extremity Uninvolved extremity	
Bad arm (or leg)	Weak arm (or leg) Affected arm (or leg)	Involved extremity Nonfunctional extremity
Client did	Client performed Client demonstrated Client participated	Client engaged Client worked on
Client said Client told	Client stated Client reported Client expressed	Client articulated Client indicated Client verbalized
Client walked	Client ambulated Client performed functional mobility	
Gave client (i.e., buttonhook)	Client was issued Client was provided	
Client took off (i.e., shirt)	Client doffed	
Client put on (i.e., pants)	Client donned	
Showed client Helped client	Client was instructed Client was taught Client was educated	Client was trained Recommended (i.e., a device or technique)
Made (i.e., splint)	Fabricated Customized	
Changed	Modified Adapted Customized	Updated Revised
Looked at (i.e., for safety or ability)	Observed Assessed Reassessed	Evaluated Examined
Put	Positioned Set up	
Upper extremity dressing Lower extremity dressing	Upper body dressing Lower body dressing	

When first learning to write client observations, it is hard to decide what to include and what to leave out. At first, it is best to include too much data, rather than take a chance on omitting something important. As your observational skills become more refined, it will become second nature to include all of the important data and instinctively eliminate the "fluff." Then, the "O" section of your notes will begin to be more professional and concise. Here is a client observation written by an inexperienced OTA. In an effort to include all of the necessary data, this note is too "wordy."

> **O:** *Client was seen in rehab gym for hot pack and Ⓡ UE strengthening. Client first had a hot pack applied to Ⓡ shoulder for 20 minutes. After the hot pack came off, client was asked to clasp hands together and raise arms above head 30X. Pt was then instructed to cross her midline and touch her opposite shoulder with Ⓡ UE. Client required six rest periods for completion. Client completed tasks Ⓘ. Client was then introduced to weight and pulley system. Client was asked to specify how much weight she thought she could do. She responded with 5#. Client did 30 reps of the pulley system with 5# in shoulder flexion to strengthen her rotator cuff to decrease the probability of dislocating her shoulder again.*

An OTA with more experience might have written a more concise note:

> **O:** *Client participated in 50-minute OT session in rehab gym to prevent further Ⓡ shoulder dislocation. Hot pack applied to Ⓡ shoulder for 20 min followed by the following Ⓡ UE strengthening exercises for rotator cuff:*
> - *Ⓑ clasped hand shoulder flexion and extension x 30 repetitions*
> - *Horizontal adduction Ⓡ hand to Ⓛ shoulder x 30 repetitions*
> - *6 rest periods were needed to complete above exercises.*
> - *Ⓡ shoulder flexion using pulleys with 5# wt. x 30 repetitions*

You will notice, however, that there is still another problem with this note. It sounds like a physical therapy note rather than an occupational therapy note. This note needs to have functional components added, although they do not have to be in the "O." A statement from the client in the "S" about what she is unable to do with an injured rotator cuff and a statement in the "A" and/or "P" indicating functional problems/goals would suffice to make it a good occupational therapy note. Notice that being more concise means knowing what information can be omitted without compromising the quality of the observation.

It is possible to be **too** succinct, thereby omitting necessary information. For example, consider the following "O" from an inpatient occupational therapy session.

> **O:** *Client seen bedside for instruction in dressing techniques.*

This "O" does not provide much information. When additional information is added, we learn quite a bit more about the session with this client:

> **O:** *Client participated in 45-minute OT session bedside for skilled instruction in dressing techniques. Client exhibited some difficulty with sequencing and attempted to don slacks before underwear. Client also required min verbal cues to attend to Ⓛ side to place Ⓛ arm in shirt sleeve. Fine motor skills were WFL to manage buttons, but moderate Ⓐ was needed to line up and fasten buttons properly 2° inattention to detail.*

It is a matter of carefully balancing the need to be complete when writing the "O" with the need to be concise. In Worksheet 7-3, you will have an opportunity to make an observation more concise, without losing any of its informational content.

This chapter has explained the basic components for writing the objective part of your SOAP note. The "O" section requires proper organization and a succinct summary describing what skilled occupational therapy services were provided in what setting. It is important that you use professional language and not duplicate services of another discipline. To make your documentation even better, there are other factors to consider when writing the "O" part of an occupational therapy note. The next chapter will provide you with more tips for writing the "O" and making your notes more accurate, professional, and complete. Remember, as you practice writing and gain clinical experience, your documentation skills will become much easier.

Worksheet 7-1
Organizing the "O" With Categories

Consider the following chronological observation:

> *Child engaged in 60-minute OT session in daycare setting to work on reach/grasp/release and feeding skills. With min (A) for facilitation of movement at elbow, child demonstrated ability to use (L) UE to reach, grasp, and release 5 objects with 1-2 verbal cues per object and used (R) UE to stabilize self for unsupported sitting at table. Child was able to feed self (I) c̄ ~50% spillage, but demonstrated significant limitations in chewing action c̄ ~3 rotary chews & swallowing ~90% of food without chewing. Child required verbal cues throughout session to maintain attention to task. Child wore soft spica thumb splint for entire session*

How would you divide this information into categories to make it more organized and easier to read? Choose 3 to 4 categories and redistribute the information above into the categories you have chosen.

Morreale, M. J., & Borcherding, S. (2013). *The OTA's guide to documentation: Writing SOAP notes (3rd ed.).* Thorofare, NJ: SLACK Incorporated.

Worksheet 7-2
Using Professional Language

Rewrite the following sentences to make them sound more concise and professional.

1. Client was asked by OTA to put on a bathrobe and slippers to determine client's ability to perform dressing. Client needed three verbal cues to tie the belt and two verbal cues to figure out which was the right slipper and which was the left. She walked from her bed to a chair using a rolling walker and OTA had to give her CGA because client was unsteady. OTA propped up client with pillows so client's bad arm would be supported and elevated and she would no longer lean to the right while sitting in the chair.

2. Client said he has pain and numbness in his Ⓡ hand due to his carpal tunnel syndrome. A splint called a cock-up splint was made to support his wrist and help decrease his symptoms. The client practiced putting on and taking off his splint. Client was able to put the splint on and remove it independently.

Morreale, M. J., & Borcherding, S. (2013). *The OTA's guide to documentation: Writing SOAP notes (3rd ed.)*. Thorofare, NJ: SLACK Incorporated.

Worksheet 7-3
Being More Concise

Revise the following treatment observations to make the note complete but more concise and professional.

O: *Pt seen 30 minutes in his hospital room for BADLs. Client ambulated ~36 inches to shower stall with SBA for safety. Client instructed to complete shower while sitting. Client performed shower with SBA to manage IV line. Client able to wash upper and lower body Ⓘ and dry entire body after completing shower. Client required ~20 minutes to complete shower. Client then ambulated ~36 inches to chair and sat. Client needed verbal cues to remain seated while donning underwear and pants. Client able to dress UE Ⓘ and lower body p̄ verbal cues for sitting. Client demonstrated good sitting balance, but needed SBA for standing balance. Following shower, client stated he would like to take a nap. Client walked to his bed with SBA and was assisted back into bed.*

Morreale, M. J., & Borcherding, S. (2013). *The OTA's guide to documentation: Writing SOAP notes (3rd ed.).* Thorofare, NJ: SLACK Incorporated.

Chapter 8

Tips for Writing a Better "O"

This chapter contains additional tips to improve your clinical reasoning and refine your documentation skills. By incorporating these principles, your notes will appear more professional and complete, and you will be more likely to comply with third-party payer guidelines.

Focus on Function

Make certain that occupation is integral to the note. In an intervention session devoted to self-care activities, function is obvious. In other circumstances, **function must be addressed separately** in order to justify skilled occupational therapy. Sessions where physical agent modalities (PAMs) are used or sessions devoted to treating client factors such as strength, range of motion, and endurance all need function emphasized in the treatment note. For example, although the following note is an observation of a session that was devoted to client factors, it contains a statement about the functional intent of the exercises.

O: _Client worked on_ Ⓛ _UE AROM and strengthening exercises at bedside_ **in order to regain ability to dress self**_. Following skilled instruction, client performed self-ranging exercises sitting on EOB c̄ stand-by_ Ⓐ _for balance and verbal instructions to correct errors. Client was verbally cued X5 to reach higher with_ Ⓛ _UE during shoulder flexion AROM to attain range needed for_ **donning a pullover shirt**.

Write From the Client's Point of View and Avoid Mentioning Yourself

The focus of good professional writing should be on the client and not the OTA (Kettenbach, 2009). Turn your sentences around so that the client is the subject of your sentence.

Rather than saying: _"The OTA put the client's shoes on for him."_
You might say: _"Client_ Ⓓ _in donning shoes."_

Rather than saying: _"OTA instructed the client and family in energy conservation techniques."_
You might say: _"Client and family were instructed in energy conservation techniques and demonstrated understanding by performing correctly."_

Morreale MJ, Borcherding S.
The OTA's Guide to Documentation:
Writing SOAP Notes, Third Edition (pp 69-78).
© 2013 SLACK Incorporated.

Focus on the Client's Response to the Intervention Provided Rather Than on What the OTA Did

Rather than saying: *"Client was reminded about hip precautions."*
You might say: *"Attempting to don shoes, client required 3 verbal cues to keep hip in correct alignment."*

Rather than saying: *"Client was asked orientation questions pertaining to the time of day."*
You might say: *"When verbally cued to look at watch, client was unable to correctly identify time."*

Rather than saying: *"Client reminded to relax when interacting with sales clerk."*
You might say: *"When interacting with sales clerk, client exhibited anxiety and required 2 verbal cues to relax."*

Rather than saying: *"Child was asked a series of yes/no questions"*
You might say: *"Child responded correctly to 2 out of 10 yes/no questions."*

De-emphasize the Treatment Media

In order to improve a client's performance skills, OTAs often use various media, such as exercise equipment, worksheets, or other preparatory activities that will help the client reach functional goals. However, when recording observations of those types of treatment activities, the OTA should de-emphasize the media used and focus instead on the performance skills being addressed. For example, an inexperienced OTA might write the following:

"Client worked on placing pegs into a pegboard."

This sentence may accurately describe what a casual observer would see. However, as a trained professional, the OTA needs to look beyond the media used and see what the client was really accomplishing. The treatment media used here are pegs and a pegboard, but what is the performance skill? Placing pegs into a pegboard is not a practical skill a client needs in order to be able to care for himself. However, the performance skill practiced during this activity may well be crucial to achieving independence. Suppose the OTA had written:

"Client worked on tripod pinch using pegs and a pegboard."

Notice that in this example the OTA did not simply add the performance skill to the statement *"Client worked on placing pegs into a pegboard to increase tripod pinch"* but actually turned the sentence around so that the tripod pinch received the emphasis and the treatment media was mentioned only for clarification. Suppose that the OTA had written:

"Client worked on tripod pinch in order to be able to grasp objects needed for ADL tasks."

In this case, mention of the media becomes optional. The OTA might also have written:

"Client worked on tripod pinch using pegs and a pegboard in order to be able to grasp objects needed for ADL tasks."

Which of the three preceding examples do you think best describes the skilled occupational therapy instruction that is occurring in this treatment session? This may seem like a minor distinction, but it is very important in demonstrating the need for skilled occupational therapy and the emphasis on functional outcomes in therapy.

One of the most common errors that inexperienced OTAs make is focusing on the media used rather than on the performance skill that is being improved by use of the media. Consider this OTA's observation:

Client seen 30 minutes in rehab gym for standing balance activities. Client stood to walker with min Ⓐ for balloon toss. Client used Ⓡ UE to hit balloon and was able to reach to Ⓡ and Ⓛ sides approximately 7 out of 10 tries. Activity was continued for 3 minutes. Client requested rest-break and sat for 30 seconds. Client then stood with mod Ⓐ to walker and hit balloon with Ⓛ UE for 3 minutes. Client was able to hit balloon approximately 6 out of 10 times and spontaneously switched to Ⓡ hand x2 when balloon was to her far right. Client sat for another break and to switch activities. Client stood CGA to toss beanbags with Ⓡ hand for 4 minutes. Client scored 240 points with Ⓡ hand by throwing beanbags at target. Once all beanbags were thrown, client sat for a 30-second break. Client stood with CGA for balance to toss beanbags with Ⓛ hand for 3½ minutes. Client scored 150 points with Ⓛ hand by throwing beanbags at scoring target. Once all beanbags were thrown, client sat and session was ended.

When this note is rewritten to focus on the performance skills instead, notice the significant difference in professionalism in the way the note reads:

Client engaged in 30-minute OT session in rehab gym to work on dynamic and static standing balance activities needed for ADL and IADL tasks. Pt. stood to walker with mod Ⓐ for dynamic standing balance necessary for Ⓘ showering using a balloon toss activity. Client held walker with Ⓛ hand and used Ⓡ UE to reach both Ⓡ and Ⓛ sides approximately 7/10 attempts. Client sustained activity for 3 minutes continuously and then took a 30-second rest break. Client stood to walker again with mod Ⓐ for 3 minutes of continuous activity involving weight shifting and balance required in balloon tossing. Client demonstrated ability to reach to Ⓡ and Ⓛ sides to reach for moving object approximately 6/10 times. Client demonstrated ability to spontaneously shift weight 2 times to reach object. Client took 30-second rest break before next activity. Client stood to walker for 4 minutes of dynamic balance activity with CGA to perform beanbag toss activity with target, then sat for 30-second rest. Client stood again with CGA for 3 1/2 minutes of continuous dynamic balance activity.

Make It Very Clear That You Were not Just a Passive Observer in the Session

This will be a critical factor in reimbursement. OTAs do not get paid to just **watch** a client do something. To demonstrate that the skill of an occupational therapy practitioner is needed, you must be **actively involved** in intervention, such as assessing or modifying the activity; otherwise it will be considered unskilled.

Rather than saying: *"Client compensated for shoulder flexion by leaning forward with whole body during prehension activities."*
You might say: *"Client required skilled instruction to avoid compensation at the shoulder during prehension activities."*
Rather than saying: *"Client performed home exercise program."*
You might say: *"Home exercise program was observed for accurate movement patterns and updated to accommodate for progress."*

Although You Will Assess the Information You Observed and Make a Professional Judgment About It, Avoid Judging the Client

Rather than saying: *"Client was compliant." or "Client was cooperative."*
You might say: *"Client demonstrated ability to follow 3-step directions and sequence WFL."*
Rather than saying: *"Child was difficult to treat today because she did not want to use a built-up spoon for self-feeding"*
You might say: *"Child required four verbal prompts to pick up and use built-up spoon to begin self-feeding."*

When working with a client who exhibits difficult personality traits or behavior, or whose opinions or values you do not agree with, it is easy to judge the client and to reflect your judgments in the "O." However, you must be careful to maintain your professional attitude and avoid personal or emotional bias. Below is an example of a note written by an OTA who was experiencing a difficult client situation. The client "went off on" the OTA. The client refused to get out of bed, lied about having already performed grooming tasks, threw her toothpaste on the floor, refused to brush her teeth or comb her hair, and cursed at the OTA. In spite of all this, the OTA wrote an observation that was nonjudgmental of the client:

Client initially declined therapy, but after max encouragement demonstrated Ⓘ supine → sit on EOB c̄ good dynamic sitting balance to perform grooming. Client expressed frustration regarding her illness by saying several profane words and throwing item on floor. Client demonstrated ability to use reacher Ⓘ to retrieve toothpaste tube from floor. Client Ⓘ brushed hair and teeth with use of bedside table and set-up.

Worksheet 8-1
De-emphasizing the Treatment Media

Rewrite the following statements to concisely emphasize the skilled occupational therapy that is actually occurring in the intervention session.

1. Client played a game of catch using bilateral UEs to facilitate grasp and release patterns.

2. Resident put dirt into pot to halfway point, added seedling, and filled remainder of pot with dirt, which was transferred by cup. Resident completed three more pots while standing 8 minutes before requiring a 5-minute rest. Resident then resumed standing position for approximately 5 minutes to water completed pots.

3. Client painted some picture frames in crafts group to be able to see that she could do something successfully.

4. Child traced around a can to make a circle and then cut out the circle to work on his visual-motor skills. He also drew a face in the circle and glued it onto a paper bag to make a puppet.

Morreale, M. J., & Borcherding, S. (2013). *The OTA's guide to documentation: Writing SOAP notes (3rd ed.)*. Thorofare, NJ: SLACK Incorporated.

Be Specific About Assist Levels

1. **Note what *specific aspect* of the activity the client needed assistance or cues to perform**. For example:
   - *Veteran doffed night garment with min Ⓐ **to untie strings on back***.
   - *Pt. able to sequence steps to prepare cup of tea but required verbal cue **to turn off stove***.
   - *Child needed hand-over-hand assist **for accuracy** when cutting with scissors*.
   - *Client required two verbal cues **to sit down** in order to doff hosiery*.
   - *Consumer able to follow bus schedule with min verbal cues **to identify correct time***.
   - *Patient stand → w/c using a standard walker with CGA and min verbal cues **to bring walker completely back to w/c***.
   - *Infant able to roll supine to prone with min tactile cues at hip **to initiate movement***.
   - *Client required mod Ⓐ **to follow total hip precautions** while using long-handled sponge for washing lower legs and feet*.
   - *Student required min verbal cues **to recall the numbers** needed to open combination lock on locker*.

2. **Describe the exact *type* and *amount* of assistance that the client needed**. It is essential that you note both the **type** of assistance and **how much** assistance the client needed to perform the activity. For example, writing *"Client required assistance to don upper and lower body garments,"* does not give someone reading your note the full picture. Did the client require minimal assistance, moderate assistance, or maximal assistance? Perhaps the client was able to perform the task by himself but needed contact guard or stand-by assistance for balance or safety. Did the client require hand-over-hand assistance to hold an item or move an extremity in order to perform the task? How much assistance was required to maintain attention, balance, stabilization, or upright posture? Did the client use compensatory methods or adaptive devices? Were there safety issues or problems with performance skills, client factors, or performance patterns? In addition, be sure to indicate that the client needed assist rather than labeling the client as an assist level. For example, state *"Client **required** min assist for standing balance when shaving at sink,"* rather than *"Client **was** min assist for standing balance when shaving at sink."*
   - *Resident needed max Ⓐ X 2 to transfer from w/c to bed*.
   - *Child required intermittent tactile cues at hip and upper torso to maintain upright posture 10 minutes when seated at desk*.
   - *Toddler required hand-over-hand assist to hold and push toy vacuum with Ⓡ hand*.
   - *Client required SBA for balance when standing to pull up and fasten pants*.
   - *Patient required mod Ⓐ to stabilize Ⓛ elbow in extended position for weightbearing while shaving at sink*.
   - *Client required min Ⓐ to place sock on sock aid and then mod Ⓐ to position device properly and pull up sock on Ⓡ LE*.

   If supervision was needed due to particular safety concerns, mental health issues, or cognitive impairment, you should clearly indicate the reason and level of supervision needed. Did the client require distant supervision within line of sight or only occasional monitoring when interacting with peers or completing an ADL, worksheet, project, etc.? Perhaps, instead, the client required close supervision within arm's length for problem solving, sequencing, or safety when using hazardous materials. Did the client require any cues? If so, how many cues and what kind—physical, verbal, auditory, or visual?
   - *Student required verbal cues every 30 seconds to attend to task when copying 10 vocabulary words from blackboard*.
   - *Client required close supervision for use of sharps during crafts group*.
   - *Resident required a visual cue (red line) in order to locate all of the words on the left side of the page*.
   - *Student required line-of-sight supervision during recess in order to monitor aggressive tendencies*.
   - *Resident required three verbal cues for proper hand placement when transferring bed ↔ commode*.
   - *Client required five verbal cues in order to verbalize two positive statements about herself*.
   - *Patient required close supervision for safe handling of hot foods when cooking*.
   - *Client needed a timer in order to take a shower and wash hair in <15 minutes*.
   - *Child required close supervision to avoid putting objects in mouth when making a macaroni necklace*.

In trying to be concise, sometimes inexperienced OTAs make the mistake of writing an "O" that contains only a list of actions with assist levels. Although this is a common error, it is **incorrect**. Simply writing a list of activities or assist levels does not demonstrate that skilled OT is being provided. Consider this OTA's observation:

> *Client was seen for 1 hour in the shower room to ↑ activity tolerance and improve balance during showering in order to prepare for discharge in one week.*
> *Client OX4.*
> *Client min Ⓐ with verbal cues to sit in w/c to doff hosiery and to dry off LE.*
> *Client spontaneously rinsed soap off hands before gripping grab bar while showering.*
> *Client used walker going to and coming from shower room.*
> *Client tolerated standing Ⓘ during entire shower.*
> *Client instructed in home showering.*

Now look at the same observation rewritten in a more useful format:

> *Client participated in 1-hour BADL session in the shower room to ↑ activity tolerance and improve balance during showering in order to prepare her for Ⓘ and safe showering after discharge in 1 week.*
> ***Mobility**: Pt. ambulated to/from shower room Ⓘ and safely with the aid of a standard walker to provide stability in shower room while dressing/undressing.*
> ***Cognition**: Client oriented X 4.*
> ***BADLs**: Client needed min Ⓐ and 2 verbal cues to sit down in order to doff hosiery and to dry LEs safely. During shower, client spontaneously rinsed soap off hands prior to gripping grab bar s̄ verbal cues. Client tolerated standing Ⓘ ~5 minutes during shower s̄ SOB. Skilled instruction provided in safe technique to use in her home shower stall and recommendations given re: grab bar placement.*

Table 8-1 provides suggestions for documenting client transfers accurately and professionally in the "O" part of your SOAP note.

Use Standardized Terminology to Describe and Grade Your Treatment Activities

It is very important to qualify and quantify the complexity level of the activities that your clients engage in. Consider the activity demands to determine and document how your interventions are graded and adapted. Often, even a very basic task has gradable components. For example, the activity requirements are easier for donning slip-on shoes rather than shoes that require tying. Perhaps, instead, the client uses shoes with hook and loop closure or elastic laces. Pants with elastic waistbands are easier to don than pants that require fastening with a button and zipper. Did the client don a button-down shirt or a pullover shirt and a front closure, back closure, or pullover bra? Try to be as specific as possible with the activity demands. For an observation noted as *"Client required assistance to don upper and lower body garments,"* it would be better to say:

> *While sitting on EOB, client required min Ⓐ and three verbal cues to place elastic waist pants over weak lower extremity with use of reacher. Client then donned slip-on shoes with supervision and verbal cue for task initiation. CGA required for balance to stand and pull up pants. Resident donned front closure bra with min Ⓐ to fasten. Client donned pullover sweater with verbal cue to identify front/back of sweater.*

Another example would be a home management task such as preparing lunch. Instead of saying, *"Client SBA in preparing lunch,"* it would be better to describe the type or complexity of lunch that the client prepared, such as:

> *Meal preparation skills assessed. Client required SBA to prepare a simple one-step microwave frozen meal. Client able to read and follow package directions, open package, and program time correctly but required two verbal cues to use potholder for safe handling of hot food.*

Table 8-2 presents some suggestions and examples for grading and describing kitchen tasks for documentation. You may come up with other categories. For each meal preparation task that your client performs, consider the activity demands such as number of steps involved, level of complexity, performance skills, and client factors required. Note if the task involves safety considerations, sequencing and organizational skills, reading directions, interpreting pictures or diagrams, opening packages, measuring, using cooking utensils or appliances, clean up, and time management.

Table 8-1	Documenting Transfers	
Steps for Documenting Transfers	**Examples**	
1. Specify the occupational therapy skill provided during the transfer	Assessment of transfer technique Assessment of DME needs Transfer training Client education Instruction in use of tub bench, commode, etc.	Instruction in compensatory techniques Instruction in weightbearing/medical precautions Family/caregiver education Safety training Increase activity tolerance
2. Relate to occupational performance and differentiate from other disciplines such as PT	…transfer training in order to bathe ① using tub bench …instruction in compensatory transfer techniques in order to adhere to total hip precautions when toileting …instruction in safe techniques for car transfers	
3. Specify the surface from which the client began the transfer	**From:** standing position edge of bed wheelchair (type) Geri chair therapy mat tub bench shower chair bathtub shower stall	toilet (high or low) commode stool chair (with or without arms, low or high, wheeled) sofa floor car classroom desk
4. Specify the surface to which the client transferred	**To:** (same as above)	
5. List any assistive devices, adaptive techniques, or environmental modifications utilized	**Using:** bed rails trapeze grab bar raised toilet seat commode frame over toilet standard walker	rolling walker quad cane cane sliding board Hoyer Lift holding onto furniture, counter, sink, etc.
6. List the type and amount of physical and verbal assistance required	Level of physical assist (e.g. mod, max) Number of persons assisting (x1, x2) Amount of verbal, visual, or tactile cues	
7. List the part of the task that required assistance	…to lock w/c brakes …to remove lap tray …to adhere to total hip precautions …for balance …to flex trunk/lean forward …to position lower extremities …to position walker, sliding board, etc. …for hand placement …for sequence of steps	…for redirection to task …to scoot to the edge of the bed, w/c, etc. …to promote weight shift …to prevent knee from buckling …to stabilize lower extremity …to push up from sitting …to control pacing when returning to sit …to manage IV pole …to manage catheter bag
8. Other considerations, if not already noted	Stable versus unstable surface Cognition (e.g., attention, problem solving) Specific safety concerns/impulsivity Ability to remember and adhere to weightbearing or other precautions Vital signs/medical considerations such as oxygen level, blood pressure, pulse, telemetry, IV lines, etc. Fear or anxiety Endurance/shortness of breath Understanding of process Demonstration required Carryover of technique Number of trials	

Worksheet 8-2
Being Specific About Assist Levels

When noting assist levels in your observation, it is not enough to note only the level of assistance required. You must also note the **specific aspect** of the task that required assistance and the **type and amount** of assistance provided. For example:

*Resident donned pants **with min Ⓐ to pull up over hips.***

*Student able to operate power w/c **using 2-lb wrist weight to minimize Ⓡ UE tremors and control joystick.***

*When observed for proper technique, foster parent required **four verbal cues to feed infant more slowly** in order to promote better swallowing of puréed foods.*

*Client propelled w/c from room to OT clinic but required **mod verbal cues to avoid running into other clients.***

Rewrite the statements below to indicate a **part** of the task that required assistance. Since you have not seen the client, you cannot really know what part required assistance. In the usual world of professional behavior, fabricating information is fraud, so please realize that the client you are about to imagine is just a creative exercise for learning purposes. For this exercise, you will create a client in your mind and imagine that client performing the task. As you watch your client in your mind, note what aspect of the task required assistance and modify the statements below accordingly to make them more specific.

1. Client supine → sit with min Ⓐ; bed → w/c with mod Ⓐ.

2. Client required SBA in transferring w/c ↔ toilet.

3. Client retrieved garments from low drawers with min Ⓐ.

4. Brushing hair required max Ⓐ.

5. Client completed dressing, toileting, and hygiene with min Ⓐ.

Morreale, M. J., & Borcherding, S. (2013). *The OTA's guide to documentation: Writing SOAP notes (3rd ed.).* Thorofare, NJ: SLACK Incorporated.

Table 8-2
Graded Levels of Meal Preparation

- Obtain a snack (get yogurt or fruit from refrigerator, cheese and crackers)
- Simple cold meal preparation (cereal and milk, sandwich)
- Cold meal preparation involving safety/tool use (salad, tuna fish)
- Microwave snack or meal (popcorn, frozen dinner, soup)
- Toaster or toaster oven (toast, waffles, frozen pizza)
- Simple stovetop task (tea, soup)
- Min complex stovetop task (grilled cheese, pudding, scrambled eggs)
- Mod complex stovetop task (tacos, macaroni and cheese)
- Complex meal preparation (following a recipe; 2-, 3-, 4-course meal)

You can apply these principles to other activities such as home management tasks. Consider the activity demands of light household chores (folding towels, wiping a table, dusting) versus heavy household chores (mopping a floor, washing windows, or changing sheets). Also, if the client uses an ambulation device or wheelchair for mobility or safety during functional tasks, the specific type of device should be noted. While not an all-inclusive list, some types of ambulation devices and wheelchairs are listed as follows:

- Crutches
- Single-point cane
- Quad cane
- Hemi-walker
- Standard walker
- Rolling walker
- Platform walker
- Standard wheelchair
- Power wheelchair
- Bariatric wheelchair
- Sip and puff wheelchair

Remember that as an OTA, you are not issuing ambulation devices or simply instructing the client in ambulation or gait training. That is most likely considered physical therapy and would be duplication of services or possibly beyond your scope of practice. Rather, in occupational therapy, your focus is on **safe functional mobility for specific occupational tasks**. You might say:

- *Resident required min Ⓐ to get clothes out of closet while standing with rolling walker.*
- *Using crutches, student required min verbal cues and CGA to stand and use reacher to obtain items on bottom of locker.*
- *Child was able to safely use platform walker to navigate in bathroom, transfer on/off toilet, and stand to manage clothing for toilet hygiene.*
- *Client needed CGA for balance to stand with quad cane and load dishwasher.*

Document Use of Physical Agent Modalities Properly

OTs and OTAs often use PAMs as a means to improve client factors such as decreasing pain and edema, increasing passive and active ROM, and promoting wound healing. However, the AOTA asserts that a PAM is not considered to be occupational therapy unless linked specifically to occupational performance and incorporated into a more comprehensive treatment program (AOTA, 2012). Therefore, it is important to document how **the PAM prepares or enables the client to perform specific functional tasks**. In addition, since another OT or OTA might be treating the client in your absence, it is necessary to document the proper parameters for the modality to ensure accuracy, safety, and consistent follow through. The OT determines which PAMs are appropriate for the client's intervention plan and supervises any modalities that the OTA administers (AOTA, 2012). Realize that various states may have strict rules or restrictions regarding the use of PAMs by OTs or OTAs. It is essential that occupational therapy practitioners who supervise or administer PAMs have service competency, follow ethical guidelines, and always adhere to state laws and regulations (AOTA, 2012). Use Table 8-3 as a guide when documenting the use of PAMs.

Table 8-3
Documenting Physical Agent Modalities
Physical Agent Modality Checklist for Documentation
Part and Place: Indicate where modality was applied on the body (e.g., right shoulder, left dorsal wrist).
Parameters: Note settings such as time, temperature, intensity, etc.
Positioning Considerations: Note any special position of client or extremity (e.g., limb placed in a stretched position, digits wrapped in flexion, active exercise while modality applied, etc.)
Purpose/Preparation: Specify the client factor, functional task, or therapeutic goal that is being addressed (e.g., pain relief, ROM, ADLs, scar management, etc.). Relate to occupational performance.
Problems/Progress: Describe client tolerance to the treatment, any modifications required, and any progress or problems pertaining to the modality.

Here are some examples for recording the use of PAMs:

- *Hot pack applied 20 minutes to Ⓡ wrist to ↓ pain and stiffness to enable performance of kitchen tasks (i.e., lifting pots, cutting vegetables). Wrist placed in flexed position for stretch and client's skin checked at 5 minutes and upon removal of hot pack. No problems noted and client reported her wrist "feels much looser after the heat." Client then was instructed in use of an ergonomic knife to chop vegetables, and she demonstrated ability to lift a small pan containing 2 cups water without report of pain.*

- *US applied to reduce pain and ↑ AROM Ⓛ shoulder to enable return to work. Pt. supine while continuous ultrasound applied 5 minutes to Ⓛ shoulder at 1MHz and 1.5 W/cm². Pt. then worked on pulleys and job simulation task of stacking 1- and 2-lb. cans on shelves c̄ Ⓛ UE. Pt. demonstrated ability to flex Ⓛ shoulder 158° and stack 30 cans without report of pain. Pt. also demonstrated ability to lift and carry 10-lb grocery bag 40 feet X 4.*

- *Fluidotherapy applied 110° for 15 minutes to Ⓛ wrist and hand to ↑ grasp and release for precision tool use. During fluidotherapy treatment client performed wrist and hand AROM exercises. Client then worked on job-related tasks and successfully used needle nose pliers to bend wire and place nails when hammering.*

HELPFUL HINT
Good documentation is based on accurate observation, which is based on knowing what to look for. For an experienced professional, this becomes second nature. For an OTA student, it is helpful to review the lists in this manual and to check your observations against what your supervising therapist observed during the intervention session to be sure you are noticing the items that matter most.

You have now completed the "O" part of your note. In this section, it is extremely important that you focus on function, de-emphasize the treatment media, and make it clear that skilled occupational therapy services were provided. Observe and assess the client's performance skills and client factors without judging the individual. Succinctly and accurately describe the complexity level and specific activity demands that your interventions entail, along with the amount and type of assistance needed. You will now move on to Chapter 9, which addresses the third section of the SOAP note—the assessment.

Chapter 9

Writing the "A"—Assessment

The third part of the note is the **ASSESSMENT**. This section consists of the occupational therapy practitioner's skilled appraisal of the client's progress, functional limitations, pertinent issues, and expected gains from rehabilitation. In the assessment section of the note, you will use your professional judgment to discern the meaning of the data you have presented in the "S" and "O" sections. You will also relate how these data will impact on the client's ability to benefit from occupational therapy and engage in meaningful occupations.

For example, during the intervention session, you may have observed that the client does not attend to the left side. Perhaps you observed that he only ate food on the right side of his meal tray and he couldn't find the toothpaste tube or brush on the bathroom counter. You will note both the problem (left neglect) and the areas of occupation in which it is a problem (BADL tasks). In your assessment, to address the impact of this deficit, you might write:

> *Left neglect interferes with client's ability to perform BADLs.*

In the assessment section of the note, the OTA will remark on the **3 P's**: **problems**, **progress**, and rehab **potential**. The OTA might also identify and explain inconsistencies, discuss emotional components, deliberate contexts or new issues, or present the reason that something was not implemented or achieved as planned.

Assessing the Data

To assess the data, go **sentence by sentence** through the data presented in the "S" and the "O." For each component, consider the implications for the client's engagement in meaningful occupational activities and role performance. Note what problems, progress, or rehabilitation potential you surmise. Consider the following possibilities.

Problems May Include the Following

Safety Risks

- *Safety concerns noted when child attempted to stand without locking brakes on w/c.*
- *Poor problem solving when using the stove raises safety concerns.*
- *Client's poor short-term memory limits ability to adhere to THR precautions.*
- *Client's limited coping strategies for dealing with stress raise concerns for continuing the use of narcotics.*

Morreale MJ, Borcherding S.
*The OTA's Guide to Documentation:
Writing SOAP Notes, Third Edition (pp 79-88).*
© 2013 SLACK Incorporated.

Inconsistencies Between Client Report and Objective Findings

- Although client reports anticipating no difficulty in returning to driving, her left-side neglect and visual field deficit would cause significant safety risks.
- Although the client expresses a willingness to perform ADLs, her sequencing and motor planning problems create barriers to tasks.
- Although the client expresses a desire to regain skills for return to work, he has not followed through with his home exercise program and has missed several OT appointments.
- Client verbalizes a desire to progress to the next level of responsibility but shows ↓ behavioral control when reward incentives are unavailable.
- Although student expresses a desire to improve handwriting, student has not followed through with use of thumb stabilization splint and built-up pen.

Factors Not Within Functional Limits That Can Be Influenced by Occupational Therapy Intervention

- Left-side weakness interferes with standing balance in tub.
- Left-side neglect necessitates verbal cues to attend to left side during BADL tasks.
- Continued verbal threats toward other clients indicate a need for anger management techniques.
- Right hand pain limits client's ability to perform heavy household chores.
- Lack of spatial orientation to identify letter shapes interferes with ability to learn to read.
- Increased tone in ⓡ upper limb hinders infant's ability to maintain prone on elbows ①.

Progress Remarks May Indicate One or More of the Following

Verification That the Treatment Being Provided Is Effective

- Weighted utensils decrease intention tremors by ~50% when eating.
- Spouse demonstrates good carryover in ability to transfer client safely.
- Gains in fine motor skills this week now enable child to manage finger foods ①.
- Patient has shown progress since the beginning of the week by demonstrating the ability to follow 1-step commands 80% of the time during ADL tasks.
- Client's spontaneous participation in group discussion shows good progress in developing social interaction skills.
- Infant's trunk strength is increasing as demonstrated by ability to sit unsupported for 60 seconds.
- Child's progress from 70% to 90% accuracy in shape recognition indicates good recall.
- Pt. demonstrates good carryover in care and use of protective splint.

Statements That Previous Goals Have Been Met or Changed

- STG #2 (Transfer to toilet with min assist) met this week.
- STG #3 upgraded to "Stand at sink for 10 minutes to perform grooming tasks c̄ SBA."
- STG #4 changed to "Initiate conversation with peer during craft group."

Reasons for the Lack of Progress

- Student has become more dependent in transfers this week 2° medication change resulting in ↑ tone in Ⓑ LEs.
- Patient has become more dependent in ADL tasks this week due to acute infection.
- Client has been unable to follow through with home program due to death of spouse.
- Resident has had increased difficulty self-feeding this week 2° wound in dominant hand.

Potential for Success in Rehabilitation

- *Resident's intact sensation and presence of voluntary movement demonstrate good rehabilitation potential.*
- *Client's ability to recognize stressors shows good potential to change maladaptive coping strategies.*
- *Student's improvement from 50% to 60% accuracy with typing words using mouthstick indicates good potential to meet goals stated in IEP.*
- *Patient's ability to recall and demonstrate 3/3 total hip precautions shows good potential to follow hip precautions after discharge.*

> **HELPFUL HINT**
>
> The assessment section demonstrates your clinical reasoning as an OTA and is the "heart" of your note. If you could write only 6 lines, the assessment section of your note would contain the 6 lines you would choose.

Assessing Factors Not Within Functional Limits

Every note does not necessarily reflect **progress** and/or rehabilitation **potential**. However, most notes do indicate **problem** areas. This is because the problems are what limit occupational performance and necessitate client treatment. The most common problem area that the OTA assesses is the impact of an underlying limiting factor such as a performance skill or client factor that is deficient. Of course, other areas delineated in the *Framework–II* can also hinder the client's occupational performance, such as context and environment, performance patterns, and activity demands (AOTA, 2008b; Gateley & Borcherding, 2012). When OTA students and novice practitioners are first learning to write SOAP notes, they may find it difficult to distinguish observations from assessments. This may also result in notes that are redundant. There is a helpful formula to address a problem area that is not within functional limits. This will ensure that you are actually writing an assessment rather than an observation. State the limiting factor or circumstance at the beginning of the sentence, and then describe or relate how that factor impacts a client's functional ability in a particular area of occupation.

Underlying Limiting Factor	Functional Impact	Ability to Engage in Occupation

Look at the examples below and note how **the subject of the sentence** reflects a particular aspect of the occupational therapy domain that is not within functional limits (Gateley & Borcherding, 2012). What follows next is the negative influence it has on a specific area of occupation. This method is useful when you are first learning, but do realize there can be other ways to write assessment statements.

- Client factors:
  - *Ⓡ shoulder pain interferes with client's ability to perform sliding board transfers.*
  - *Lymphedema in right arm hinders client's ability to reach into upper kitchen cabinets.*
  - *Excessive tone in left upper extremity interferes with infant's ability to crawl.*
  - *Lack of voluntary wrist and finger extension limits child's ability to engage in developmental play activities.*
- Context and environment:
  - *The sound of sirens triggers flashbacks of client's accident and interferes with task completion at work.*
  - *Lack of elevator access impedes client's ability to enter his office.*
  - *Unavailability of public transportation limits client's ability to obtain groceries.*
  - *Poor parental supervision creates a concern for toddler's safety in the home.*
- Performance patterns:
  - *Student's routine of eating pizza and milkshakes every day for lunch contributes to his obesity, which hinders gym class participation.*
  - *Client's compulsive habit of checking locks excessively in the morning interferes with getting to work on time.*
  - *Client's dialysis schedule is a barrier to full-time employment.*
  - *Client's habit of purging after meals creates significant tension in her relationship with spouse.*

- Performance skills:
  - o *Inability to self-regulate alcoholic intake* results in difficulty maintaining employment.
  - o *Deficits in attention span* create safety concerns for riding a bicycle.
  - o *Decreased oral-motor control* interferes with child's ability to manage solid foods.
  - o *Deficits in problem solving* create a need for maximum verbal cues to perform kitchen tasks safely.
- Activity demands:
  - o *Inability to tolerate closed spaces* interferes with client's ability to use the bus.
  - o Client's *fear of germs* interferes with money handling tasks at his fast food job.
  - o Child's *tactile defensiveness* is a barrier to completing projects in school that require glue.
  - o Client's *heat intolerance* hinders ability to return to his outdoor construction job during the summer months.

Writing the Assessment

As you carefully and systematically review the material in your "S" and "O", you might find it helpful to create a quick list of things to discuss in the "A" section of your note. For example, consider the following "S" and "O":

S: *Client stated his dominant right hand "feels clumsy." He also reported difficulty with managing clothing fastenings.*

O: *Client participated in 30-minute session in OT clinic for remediation of fine motor skills and hand strength for ADLs. Client worked on three-point and lateral pinch with use of button board and clothespins. He was issued lightly resistive therapy putty and was instructed in home exercise program. Written copy of exercises also provided and client demonstrated all exercises accurately. Client was issued a buttonhook with built-up handle. He demonstrated ability to use buttonhook to fasten and unfasten small buttons Ⓘ following instruction. Client expressed willingness to continue use of buttonhook and putty at home.*

The following areas of problems/progress/potential can be identified:

- **Problems**
  - o Client is concerned regarding deficits in hand function.
  - o Client is still unable to manage fastenings independently.
- **Progress**
  - o Client is able to understand and integrate therapy tasks.
  - o Client is able to use adaptive equipment to compensate for ADL deficits.
  - o Client is willing to follow through with home program.
- **Potential**
  - o By using professional judgment, the OTA would consider the client's progress shown thus far a good indicator of rehabilitation potential. The assessment of the data can then be written as follows:

A: *Client's ability to accurately demonstrate exercises and use buttonhook indicates good rehab potential for managing fastenings and dressing Ⓘ. Client appears motivated and able to follow through with home program.*

Justifying Continued Treatment

One very useful way of justifying continued OT treatment for your client is to end the "A" with the statement, *"Client would benefit from..."* Then, based on your observations and assessment, complete the sentence with a justification of continued treatment that requires the skill of an occupational therapy practitioner rather than another discipline such as a nurse, PT, or aide. Not every OT or OTA ends the "A" in this fashion, but for purposes of learning, we will end the "A" with this method. This helps to make certain that justification for continued treatment is present in the note, and is a good way to set up the plan. As you become more proficient in writing notes and are confident that your note justifies continued treatment, you may choose to cover this material in the plan instead.

The following examples of "A" statements show justification for further skilled occupational therapy:

- *Resident would benefit from environmental cues to orient him to environment.*
- *Child would benefit from assistive technology to perform classroom tasks.*
- *Parent would benefit from further instruction in positioning child for feeding.*
- *Consumer would benefit from continued instruction in problem solving and anger management techniques needed for successful personal and social relationships.*
- *Client would benefit from continued skilled OT to improve decision-making skills and time management to ↓ maladaptive behaviors.*
- *Client would benefit from instruction in self-ranging exercises to increase left shoulder ROM for work tasks.*
- *Client would benefit from further instruction in total hip precautions in order to manage IADLs safely.*
- *Infant would benefit from activities that encourage trunk rotation to facilitate rolling over.*
- *Client would benefit from use of a reacher, sock aid, and long-handled shoe horn to minimize low back pain when performing lower body dressing.*
- *Resident would benefit from skilled instruction in sequencing of tasks to increase safety while performing toilet hygiene and bathing tasks.*
- *Client would benefit from instruction in energy conservation and work simplification techniques to perform meal preparation and clean up.*

Review the criteria for skilled occupational therapy in Chapter 3 along with the list of specialized services that occupational therapy practitioners provide. For each client, you will collaborate with the OT to consider any safety concerns or risks for secondary complications and determine what specific interventions can facilitate the client's health and occupational performance. Use your clinical reasoning to document ethically the principles and strategies used during an intervention session in justifying the continuation of skilled occupational therapy. Also, if you state that the client will benefit from further specific occupational therapy interventions, you must be prepared to follow through with this. Remember that the justification for continued occupational therapy must be reasonable and necessary for the client's condition and support the frequency, duration, and outcomes delineated in the intervention plan. If the last sentence of your "A" reads, *"Client would benefit from information on energy conservation techniques,"* do not expect the payer to approve more than one more treatment session unless you indicate that functional training and practice is required for implementation.

If this is the client's last session, complete the sentence with the OT's discharge plan for which you might have contributed to. For example:

- *Client would benefit from continued PROM provided by caregiver.*
- *Child would benefit from continued participation in recreational tennis and swimming to improve upper body strength and endurance.*
- *Client has been instructed in home safety modifications and would benefit from the installation of bathroom grab bars.*
- *Client would benefit from Meals on Wheels to eliminate need for grocery shopping.*
- *Student would benefit from continued participation in peer support group.*
- *Client would benefit from continued use of home paraffin and TENS unit PRN for pain relief.*
- *Client would benefit from a personal emergency response system at home for safety.*

Worksheet 9-1
Justifying Continued Treatment

Which of the following require the skill of an OTA?

1. _____ Administering paraffin irrelevant to occupational performance

2. _____ Instructing the client in leisure skills for stress management

3. _____ Having a client watch a video on assertiveness training without further instruction or without role-playing the techniques

4. _____ Analyzing and modifying functional tasks/activities through the provision of adaptive equipment or techniques

5. _____ Determining that the modified task is safe and effective

6. _____ Carrying out a maintenance program

7. _____ Upgrading a strengthening program

8. _____ Teaching the client to use the breathing techniques he has learned while performing his ADL activities

9. _____ Interpreting initial evaluation results and establishing the intervention plan

10. _____ Providing individualized instruction to the client, family, or caregiver

11. _____ Giving the patient a replacement piece of hook and loop fastener

12. _____ Providing specialized instruction to eliminate limitations in a functional activity

13. _____ Developing a home program and instructing caregivers

14. _____ Teaching compensatory skills

15. _____ Gait training

16. _____ Making skilled recommendations to a parent for a child's positioning and feeding

17. _____ Educating clients to eliminate safety hazards

18. _____ Presenting information handouts (such as energy conservation) without having the client perform the activity

19. _____ Routine exercise and strengthening programs

20. _____ Adding instruction in lower body dressing techniques to a current ADL program

21. _____ Teaching adaptive techniques such as one-handed shoe tying

22. _____ Helping a client in the bathroom

23. _____ Asking a client about his day

Morreale, M. J., & Borcherding, S. (2013). *The OTA's guide to documentation: Writing SOAP notes (3rd ed.)*. Thorofare, NJ: SLACK Incorporated.

Ending the Assessment

Now we can finish the assessment section of the note we began earlier:

S: *Client stated his dominant right hand "feels clumsy." He also reported difficulty with managing clothing fastenings.*

O: *Client participated in 30-minute session in OT clinic for remediation of fine motor skills and hand strength for ADLs. Client worked on three-point and lateral pinch with use of button board and clothespins. He was issued lightly resistive therapy putty and was instructed in home exercise program. Written copy of exercises also provided and client demonstrated all exercises accurately. Client was issued a buttonhook with built-up handle. He demonstrated ability to use buttonhook to fasten and unfasten small buttons Ⓘ following instruction. Client expressed willingness to continue use of buttonhook and putty at home.*

A: *Client's ability to accurately demonstrate exercises and use buttonhook indicates good rehab potential for managing fastenings and dressing Ⓘ. Client appears motivated and able to follow through with home program.* **Client would benefit from** *further instruction in adaptive equipment, compensatory techniques, and remediation of fine motor skills in order to regain Ⓘ in all ADLs.*

Here are some more examples of what the completed assessment section of your note might look like for other practice settings:

A: *Client is beginning to regain some of the independent living skills she had prior to her recent psychotic episode. Fear, isolation, and ↓ activity tolerance slow her progress and are the focus of current treatment. Client would benefit from continued skilled instruction in self-care skills as well as ↑ socialization and ↑ physical activity.*

A: *Child's poor attention span and inability to tolerate auditory stimuli limit her ability to control her classroom behavior. She would benefit from more activities to ↑ tolerance of auditory stimuli and strategies to manage self-control.*

New Information

The assessment section is **not** the place to introduce new information. Do not put anything in your "A" that has not already been discussed in the "S" or "O." If you find yourself wanting to make a statement in the "A" that is not supported by the data in your "S" or "O," ask yourself what you might have observed to support the assessment statement. Then decide whether you need to add it to your "S" or "O."

Now you can try to integrate the information in this chapter. Review the following occupational therapy note:

S: *Client stated she has difficulty moving Ⓡ UE, although she does not know why it will not move. She reported, "It really doesn't hurt. It's just tight."*

O: *Client participated in 30-minute OT session in hospital room to ↑ AROM and strength in Ⓡ shoulder, ↑ activity tolerance and dynamic standing balance in order to ↑ independence in ADL activities.*
__BADLs:__ Client was instructed on safety techniques and adaptive equipment use for toileting. Client required use of bilateral grab bars in bathroom to sit → stand safely. Client first attempted to stand while pulling on walker and one grab bar. Client was instructed on safety and the use of bilateral grab bars.
__Performance skills:__ Client sit → stand CGA for balance. Client worked on activity tolerance, dynamic standing balance, and ↑ AROM in right shoulder by moving personal hygiene items from bathroom counter to medicine cabinet for 5 minutes before needing to sit and rest 2 minutes. She then participated in activities to ↑ dynamic standing balance by pouring liquid from a pitcher while standing CGA for balance. After a 1-minute rest, client continued activities to ↑ dynamic standing balance and safety in ADL activities by pushing wheeled walker with CGA while picking up objects from the floor with a reacher.
__Client factors:__ AROM in right shoulder abduction <90°. PROM right shoulder abduction WNL.

Think about how you would assess this information. Review the suggestions given earlier in the chapter, and then organize your thoughts by identifying the problems, progress, and rehabilitation potential you see in this client's treatment session today. What **problems** and safety risks can you identify? Are there performance skills and client factors not within functional limits that occupational therapy might impact? Do you see any evidence of **progress** or rehab **potential**? What would this client benefit from? Identify problems, progress, and rehab potential using Mini Worksheet 9-2. Then compare your ideas with the suggested assessment that follows.

Mini Worksheet 9-2
Organizing Your Thoughts for Assessment

Problems

Progress

Potential

In preparing an assessment of the data in this note, two main **problem** areas can be determined: the safety of transferring to and from the toilet, and the client factors that were not within functional limits. The OTA should be particularly concerned about the safety issues, and those should be addressed first. Also, the OTA should note the rehabilitation **potential** that would help a reviewer to decide whether the client's progress is sufficient to warrant the expense of treatment.

A: *Safety concerns (impulsivity, ↓ dynamic standing balance) noted when client attempts to transfer sit → stand during toileting. Client verbalized an understanding of safety instructions and has potential to progress to independence.*

Next, the OTA should note the clinical reasoning behind devoting time to addressing client factors, considering the client's rehabilitation potential.

A: *Safety concerns (impulsivity, ↓ dynamic standing balance) noted when client attempts to transfer sit → stand during toileting. Client verbalized an understanding of safety instructions and has potential to progress to independence.* **Client's ↓ AROM in right shoulder, ↓ activity tolerance, and ↓ dynamic standing balance all interfere with ability to complete ADL tasks safely and independently.**

The OTA can then complete the assessment by justifying continued treatment.

A: *Safety concerns (impulsivity, ↓ dynamic standing balance) noted when client attempts to transfer sit → stand during toileting. Client verbalized an understanding of safety instructions and has potential to progress to independence. Client's ↓ AROM in right shoulder, ↓ activity tolerance, and ↓ dynamic standing balance all interfere with ability to complete ADL tasks safely and independently.* **Client would benefit from Ⓡ UE AROM and strengthening exercises along with continued skilled instruction on safety and energy conservation techniques.**

In this case, the OTA can address client factors in 2 different ways, both by working on ↑ AROM, strength, and activity tolerance and by teaching some energy conservation strategies.

Third-party payers often deny ongoing treatment of range of motion and strength unless significant functional gains are evident. Occupational therapy practitioners must consider the expected improvement in function versus the costs of continuing treatment. Clinical decisions must be made to determine if a home exercise program could accomplish the same results or if skilled services remain appropriate and necessary. In Chapter 10, you will see how an OTA can cost-effectively provide the proper interventions to benefit this client.

Morreale, M. J., & Borcherding, S. (2013). *The OTA's guide to documentation: Writing SOAP notes (3rd ed.).* Thorofare, NJ: SLACK Incorporated.

Worksheet 9-3
Assessing Factors Not Within Functional Limits

Use the following formula to rewrite the assessment statements and make them more effective.

Underlying Limiting Factor	Functional Impact	Ability to Engage in Occupation

For example, this statement is an observation:

Client's activity tolerance for standing at the stove was <4 minutes 2° inability to tolerate prosthesis.

It tells you the client behavior and measurable factors the OTA can observe while providing intervention. To make it into an assessment statement, you would need to change the emphasis by turning your sentence around and by adding the impact the client's standing tolerance has on her independence in cooking. Using the formula above, you might write:

Client's activity tolerance for standing with prosthesis for <4 min limits performance of kitchen tasks.

Rewrite the following statements using the formula given above.

1. Child wrote poorly due to immature pencil grasp and difficulty c̄ spatial orientation of letters.

2. Client demonstrated difficulty with balancing her checkbook due to memory and sequencing deficits.

3. Client experiencing manic episode and was unable to attend and follow directions for cooking activity.

4. Client problem solved poorly while performing lower body dressing as evidenced by multiple attempts to button pants and don socks.

Morreale, M. J., & Borcherding, S. (2013). *The OTA's guide to documentation: Writing SOAP notes (3rd ed.).* Thorofare, NJ: SLACK Incorporated.

Worksheet 9-4
Social Skills Worksheet

Your client is a middle-aged woman presently diagnosed with bipolar disorder. In a prior admission, however, she was diagnosed with schizophrenia. One of her goals is to talk to the mental health center staff about her problems rather than acting out her feelings. Today she participated in an occupational therapy social skills group with five other clients who also need help with relationship issues.

S: *Client reports that she understands the purpose of social skills group. She expressed a desire to attend all of the groups, saying that they are "fun."*

O: *Client participated in an OT group session on friendship in order to improve interpersonal skills and coping mechanisms. Client appeared unkempt, with hair not combed and shirt rumpled. Client engaged in conversation with the other clients and the facilitator, but interrupted others on 5 occasions. Client spontaneously verbalized her experiences with past friendships and her ideas of useful ways to make new friendships, but had to be redirected to the topic twice during discussion.*

What **problems** are evident in the above "S" and "O"?

What **areas of occupation** are affected by these problems?

What evidence of **progress** and/or **potential** do you see?

Write your assessment below.
  A:

Morreale, M. J., & Borcherding, S. (2013). *The OTA's guide to documentation: Writing SOAP notes (3rd ed.).* Thorofare, NJ: SLACK Incorporated.

Chapter 10

Writing the "P"—Plan

The final section of a SOAP note is the **PLAN**. In this section, you determine and set forth the specific treatment that will be used to achieve the occupational therapy goals. You will record what follow-up is required, such as what you plan to do in the client's next occupational therapy session or what must be addressed in the near future. The plan might also be a recommendation that you want the client, family, or caregiver to follow through with, such as attend a support group, install grab bars, wear a splint for work, communicate with the doctor about a particular concern, try out a home exercise program, or use an adaptive device. The plan in your SOAP note must follow the OT's intervention plan (containing long- and short-term goals, frequency and estimated duration of treatment) that was established from the initial evaluation. It should also relate to the information that you just presented in the "O" and the "A," and to your skilled assessment of what the client would benefit from.

The plan will inform the reader of your priorities regarding intervention strategies. In a contact note or a progress note, you will address any part of the plan that has not been covered in the last sentence of your assessment, *"Client would benefit from…"* You will address how often the client will be treated, how long intervention will continue, and your priorities for what you will work on next or follow up with.

> *Consumer will continue prevocational program 5 days/wk. in order to ↑ task behaviors for work such as correct use of time card and time management during breaks.*

Some facilities require that occupational therapy practitioners include goals in the "P" section. Those goals follow the OT's intervention plan and may depict the incremental steps to the established long- or short-term goals. In a practice setting such as a school system where monthly notes are written, your goal in the "P" might be what you hope to accomplish in the next month. In a skilled nursing facility, it might be your goal for the next week. In an acute care setting, it might be your goal for tomorrow.

- *Continue one hour daily sessions for 2 weeks to improve motor planning skills for dressing. By the end of next session, veteran will demonstrate the ability to identify front and back of shirt with one verbal cue.*

- *Client will continue to be seen in values clarification groups 3x/wk for 2 weeks to address low self-esteem and alcohol use. Pt. will demonstrate awareness of self-help strategies by verbalizing three alternatives to handle stress rather than drinking, within two group sessions.*

- *Continue OT for 30-minute sessions daily until discharge to facilitate improved function of affected limb for ADLs. By end of next treatment session, client will demonstrate Ⓘ in donning/doffing of splint and positioning of Ⓡ UE to minimize edema.*

- *Student will continue OT 3x weekly in order to ↑ perceptual and fine motor skills for better classroom performance. Student will be able to use loop scissors to cut a straight dotted line Ⓘ within ¼ inch 3/4 opportunities by the end of next month.*

Morreale MJ, Borcherding S.
The OTA's Guide to Documentation:
Writing SOAP Notes, Third Edition (pp 89-93).
© 2013 SLACK Incorporated.

Many facilities do not include goals in the "P" section and may only update and include goals in progress notes or reevaluation notes. You will learn how to write goals in Chapter 15. For the purpose of completing your SOAP notes at this time, we will not end the plan with a goal. Once you are proficient in goal writing, it is easy to simply add a goal statement to your plan if your facility requires it.

HELPFUL HINT

If for some reason you are not able to see your client as scheduled, the "plan" section of your note should allow another occupational therapy practitioner to continue treatment uninterrupted.

Determining the Plan

Now let us determine the plan for the note that we assessed in the last chapter. As you recall from Chapter 9, this client has deficits in safety and standing balance.

S: *Client stated she has difficulty moving ®UE, although she does not know why it will not move. She reported, "It really doesn't hurt. It's just tight."*

O: *Client participated in 30-minute OT session in hospital room to ↑ AROM and strength in ® shoulder, ↑ activity tolerance and dynamic standing balance in order to ↑ independence in ADL activities.*
__BADLs__: Client was instructed on safety techniques and adaptive equipment use for toileting. Client required use of bilateral grab bars in bathroom to sit → stand safely. Client first attempted to stand while pulling on walker and one grab bar. Client was instructed on safety and the use of bilateral grab bars.
__Performance Skills__: Client sit → stand CGA for balance. Client worked on activity tolerance, dynamic standing balance, and ↑ AROM in right shoulder by moving personal hygiene items from bathroom counter to medicine cabinet for 5 minutes before needing to sit and rest 2 minutes. She then participated in activities to ↑ dynamic standing balance by pouring liquid from a pitcher while standing CGA for balance. After a 1-minute rest, client continued activities to ↑ dynamic standing balance and safety in ADL activities by pushing wheeled walker with CGA while picking up objects from the floor with a reacher.
__Client Factors__: AROM in right shoulder abduction <90°. PROM right shoulder abduction WNL.

A: *Safety concerns (impulsivity, ↓ dynamic standing balance) noted when client attempts to transfer sit → stand during toileting. Client verbalized an understanding of safety instructions and has potential to progress to independence. Client's ↓ AROM in right shoulder, ↓ activity tolerance, and ↓ dynamic standing balance all interfere with ability to complete ADL tasks safely and independently. Client would benefit from ® UE AROM and strengthening exercises along with continued skilled instruction on safety and energy conservation techniques.*

Write your plan for this client below. Begin with a statement about how often (once or twice daily, 2x/wk, etc.) and for how long (for 3 days, for 2 weeks, for 1 month, etc.) she will receive occupational therapy. Look at the items indicated above that she would benefit from, and set your priorities.

Mini Worksheet 10-1
Determining the Plan

P:

Morreale, M. J., & Borcherding, S. (2013). *The OTA's guide to documentation: Writing SOAP notes (3rd ed.)*. Thorofare, NJ: SLACK Incorporated.

Completing the Plan

In assessing the data, the OTA has set up the plan for this note. The OTA has already justified the main intention and indicated the client's rehabilitation potential. Now the OTA needs to be specific about how often the client will be treated and for what length of time. This will reflect the frequency and duration of treatment that the OT initially established in the intervention plan. Some facilities do not restate the frequency and duration in every subsequent treatment note, but we will write the plan this way:

> **P:** *Continue OT 5X wk for 1 week...*

The OTA could have specified the length of the treatment sessions (i.e., *for 1 hr. sessions*) but chose not to do that in this particular note. Next, the OTA specifies how the treatment time will be used:

> **P:** *Continue OT 5X wk for 1 week **for skilled instruction in safe transfers and toileting**.*

Because discharge is anticipated in 1 week, the OTA must prioritize treatment time in order to implement the OT's intervention plan. As the OT has delegated treatment of this client to the OTA, the OTA might choose in this case to work on balance and energy conservation as a part of functional mobility and ADL activities. Since the OTA has already written that the client would benefit from additional AROM and strengthening exercises, there now needs to be a specific note of how these needs will be addressed:

> **P:** *Continue OT 5X wk for 1 week for skilled instruction in safe transfers and toileting. **Home program for AROM and strengthening exercises for Ⓡ shoulder will be taught**:*

This OTA has also indicated clinical reasoning in planning for discharge in advance of the discharge date. When providing feedback to the OT and recording later notes, the OTA will indicate the client's progress in learning the home program. Simply handing the client a set of printed exercises is not considered a billable service. The client's progress in learning the home program will also confirm the OTA's assessment that the client's rehabilitation potential was on target. This note is now finally complete. Here is another example of how the plan might be written for the same client.

> **P:** *Continue OT for 1 hour 5 X wk until anticipated discharge in 1 week. Client will work on safe transfers, toileting, and improving activity tolerance. Client will also be instructed in HEP to improve Ⓡ shoulder AROM and strength.*

Remember that **the time frames in the "P" section should be consistent with those established in the OT's intervention plan**. While there are often standards or norms for time frames based on the type of practice area and diagnosis, time frames vary based on payment source, facility requirements, and the client's specific circumstances (Gateley & Borcherding, 2012). When establishing the intervention plan, the OT takes those factors into account along with the physician's orders and client's past history, present status, and anticipated needs. For example, in an acute care setting, a client might be seen for just one or two occupational therapy sessions (such as for a splint, home exercise program, or equipment recommendations) or could receive therapy daily until discharge from the facility if the situation warrants it (Gateley & Borcherding, 2012). Even the length of sessions can vary from only a few minutes (such as for a client in the ICU) to 15 or 30 minutes or longer for clients who are more medically stable; whereas, clients in an inpatient rehabilitation center usually receive therapy once or twice daily for a total of 60 to 90 minutes (Gateley & Borcherding, 2012). In home care or outpatient settings, clients might only have several sessions or could receive therapy on a regular basis 2 to 3 times weekly for several weeks or longer (Gateley & Borcherding, 2012). Clients in a school setting receive occupational therapy according to what is delineated in the annual IEP, such as a monthly session or 1 or 2 times weekly. As you can see, each setting is different. Your facility will have specific requirements for what aspects of the OT's intervention plan to include in the "P" part of your note.

Worksheet 10-2
Completing the Social Skills Plan

As you recall from Chapter 9, your client is a middle-aged woman diagnosed with bipolar disorder. In a prior admission, however, she was diagnosed with schizophrenia. One of her goals is to talk to the mental health center staff about her problems rather than acting out her feelings. Today she participated in an occupational therapy social skills group with five other clients who also need help with relationship issues. The assessment's last sentence indicates some areas of intervention that might benefit this client. Now fill in the specifics of the plan.

S: *Client reports that she understands the purpose of social skills group. She expressed a desire to attend all of the groups, saying that they are "fun."*

O: *Client participated in an OT group session on friendship in order to improve interpersonal skills and coping mechanisms. Client appeared unkempt, with hair not combed and shirt rumpled. Client engaged in conversation with the other clients and the facilitator but interrupted others on 5 occasions. Client spontaneously verbalized her experiences with past friendships and her ideas of useful ways to make new friendships but had to be redirected to the topic twice during discussion.*

A: *Client's unkempt appearance, interrupting behaviors, and need for redirection to topic of conversation interfere with her ability to engage in social participation with peers. Her expressed interest in groups and her willingness to engage in conversation and share her ideas show good potential to develop relationships and to express herself verbally in place of acting out. Client would benefit from participating in groups where conversational skills are stressed along with further facilitation of attention to social cues, and from assistance with ADL activities stressing hygiene and appearance.*

P:

Morreale, M. J., & Borcherding, S. (2013). *The OTA's guide to documentation: Writing SOAP notes (3rd ed.).* Thorofare, NJ: SLACK Incorporated.

Worksheet 10-3
Completing the Plan—Additional Practice

Now try to finish the plan section for the following note. Think about what you would need to follow up with. Also consider what other specific interventions or adaptive equipment might help this client.

S: *Client stated his dominant right hand "feels clumsy." He also reported difficulty with managing clothing fastenings.*

O: *Client participated in 30-minute session in OT clinic for remediation of fine motor skills and hand strength for ADLs. Client worked on three-point and lateral pinch with use of button board and clothespins. He was issued lightly resistive therapy putty and was instructed in home exercise program. Written copy of exercises also provided and client demonstrated all exercises accurately. Client was issued a buttonhook with built-up handle. He demonstrated ability to use buttonhook to fasten and unfasten small buttons Ⓘ following instruction. Client expressed willingness to continue use of buttonhook and putty at home.*

A: *Client's ability to accurately demonstrate exercises and use buttonhook indicates good rehab potential for managing fastenings and Ⓘ dressing. Client appears motivated and able to follow through with home program. Client would benefit from further instruction in adaptive equipment, compensatory techniques, and remediation of fine motor skills in order to regain Ⓘ in all ADLs.*

P:

Morreale, M. J., & Borcherding, S. (2013). *The OTA's guide to documentation: Writing SOAP notes (3rd ed.).* Thorofare, NJ: SLACK Incorporated.

Chapter 11

Documenting Special Situations

OTAs may encounter special situations that require documentation, even if the client wasn't seen face to face or didn't receive a complete occupational therapy session. Sessions sometimes get canceled for various reasons or may involve unusual circumstances such as mishaps or unexpected events. Besides recording these situations, you should carefully document any necessary communication or follow-up regarding these events. This will ensure coordination of care and also help protect you should any legal issues arise later on. You must also record the date and time and sign the note. The following are some examples of notations for special situations.

Refusals and Cancellations

Sometimes a client might refuse or cancel occupational therapy services either completely or only for one particular session. Always document the refusal or cancellation and indicate the reason why whenever possible.

- *Client refused OT today because he felt "dizzy and nauseous." Nursing was notified.*
- *Student went on class trip and, therefore, was unable to receive OT today.*
- *Client called to cancel OT appointment because his car broke down. Appointment was rescheduled for tomorrow.*
- *Patient called and canceled his OT initial evaluation. He stated he does not want any therapy. Patient was educated regarding the reason for referral and benefits of OT, but he still refused services. MD was notified.*
- *Attempted to see client today, but client was unavailable due to medical test procedures (X-ray and MRI). Will attempt to see client again tomorrow.*
- *Father called to cancel child's appointment because child has a stomach virus.*
- *Client called crying and stated she was canceling OT today because of her agoraphobia. She reported having a severe anxiety attack this morning and was fearful of leaving her home. She also reported her medication made her "feel worse." Attempted to reassure client and advised her to contact her psychiatrist to discuss her anxiety and medication issues. Encouraged client to attend next OT session scheduled in 2 days.*

Morreale MJ, Borcherding S.
The OTA's Guide to Documentation:
Writing SOAP Notes, Third Edition (pp 95-97).
© 2013 SLACK Incorporated.

No Shows

Sometimes a client has an OT appointment and simply does not show up.

- *Pt. did not show up for appointment. Call made to pt.'s home. Pt. stated he forgot appointment. OT rescheduled for tomorrow.*
- *No show. Attempted to call pt. but no one answered the phone.*
- *Child did not show up for appointment. When parent was contacted by phone, she stated she could not get the time off from work today to bring child to OT. Appointment was confirmed for next OT session in two days.*
- *Client did not show up for appointment. Call made to client's home. Client stated he could not "get motivated" to get out of bed and get dressed due to "very depressed mood." Client did not express suicidal ideation and stated he was adhering to his medication regime. Client also stated that he realizes OT is important for his recovery and will ask his sister to bring him to tomorrow's OT session.*
- *Resident did not show up for scheduled OT session. Called nurse's station and RN stated resident wasn't feeling well this morning and was sleeping. Will attempt to see resident again this afternoon.*

Treatment Interruptions

Sometimes you are about to start an OT session or are in the middle of an intervention and the treatment gets interrupted for various reasons. Any intervention provided should be documented along with the reason for the therapy interruption.

- *Client transferred from bed to w/c with min assist. Client then stated she did not feel well and vomited. Changed client's soiled garments and notified nursing staff.*
- *Child seen in dining room for instruction in feeding skills. Five minutes into session, the physician came to take child for medical evaluation. Will attempt OT session again tomorrow for further skilled instruction in feeding.*
- *Upon arrival to OT clinic, resident stated she needed to have a bowel movement. Resident was transported back to her room and nursing staff was notified.*
- *Pt. arrived at OT visibly upset. She stated, "I can't go on. I really feel like killing myself." Attempted to calm pt. and contacted social worker, who requested COTA bring pt. to her office immediately. Pt. was then transported to social worker's office to address her emotional status.*

Medical Hold

Sometimes the client's medical condition warrants that therapy be put on hold. This may be indicated in the physician orders, by the nursing staff, by the occupational therapy practitioner's discretion, or per facility policy.

- *As per MD orders, client is on hold for therapy today due to possible blood clots in Ⓛ LE.*
- *Nursing requested that OT be deferred today due to pt.'s side effects from chemotherapy.*
- *Upon pt.'s arrival to OT clinic, pt. stated she fell yesterday on her affected Ⓡ UE. Right hand is now moderately edematous and bruised, and pt. reports severe pain. MD was immediately called. MD requested OT be put on hold until MD evaluates pt. to determine Ⓡ UE status. Pt. advised to follow up with physician ASAP.*
- *OT deferred today due to child having surgery for insertion of feeding tube.*
- *Pt. called to report he was hospitalized for two nights 2° pneumonia. OT deferred until physician's orders are received to resume OT.*
- *MD orders state client on hold 2° to psychotic episode.*

Incidents

Sometimes accidents or incidents happen no matter how careful you are. Each facility should have specific policies and procedures on how to document and handle incidents regarding staff, clients, visitors, or volunteers. Protocols are usually in place to deal with safety, security and medical issues, standard precautions, proper notification of superiors, administrative follow through, and liability issues. Typically, there are separate **incident report** forms to fill out besides the information that is recorded in the health record. Only report the actual facts. Do not embellish, guess, or make assumptions about what occurred when you are noting the incident. **Learn the exact policies and procedures in your facility so you are prepared to handle any incidents promptly and properly**.

- *Upon COTA's arrival at pt.'s room, pt. was found lying on floor crying. Nursing staff and physician were immediately notified.*
- *Upon client's arrival at OT cooking group, client suddenly picked up a pan and hit himself on the head with it, sustaining a bruise. Client was immediately removed from cooking group and taken to nurse's station for evaluation of self-inflicted injury.*
- *Client sustained a small cut to left small finger distal phalanx while cutting vegetables in cooking group. Wound cleansed and bandage applied. Nursing notified.*
- *Child became angry when told he must stay seated in his chair. He then yelled several profane words and bit COTA's hand. Child was then sent to principal's office to address inappropriate behavior.*

As an OTA, you must always be prepared to react quickly and appropriately to unexpected circumstances. Obtain the most knowledge you can regarding facility policies, emergency procedures, first aid, infection control, pertinent laws, and current occupational therapy practice so you will be prepared. When special situations and unusual circumstances do arise, you must always use professional judgment, maintain your professional demeanor, and keep the OT and other pertinent staff informed. Document in a timely manner, avoid speculation, report the facts carefully and accurately, and do what is in the client's best interest.

Chapter 12

Improving Observation Skills and Refining Your Note

In order to document intervention sessions appropriately and accurately, it is important to hone your observation skills, use clinical reasoning, organize data, and record the information methodically and professionally. As indicated in previous chapters, you will make numerous observations during a treatment session while professionally assessing the client's responses, behavior, performance skills, and other issues related to the client's condition. You will then have to document these professional observations so someone reading your note will get a clear mental picture of the client's situation and what transpired during the intervention session. If possible, jot down observations and information during the therapy session or as soon as possible. This will help you to remember pertinent facts when you later organize the information into a SOAP note. Remember that you must also properly secure and dispose of these informal notes or drafts as per HIPAA guidelines. As you gain clinical proficiency and develop your own repertoire of professional terminology, recording your observations quickly and accurately will become easier.

Tips for Improving Observation Skills

Here are some additional questions and tips to consider during client interventions. Use these suggestions to improve your observation skills and help organize information for your SOAP notes.

WHO Is Involved in the Intervention Session?

- Are family members, caregivers, or other staff present or involved in the intervention session?
- Is your client interacting with other clients?
- Is this a group activity?

WHEN Did the Intervention Session Take Place?

- Did you treat the client during a specific mealtime, during morning self-care, after dinner, during a classroom activity, group session, etc.?
- What did the client do just before your treatment session and will this impact the client's performance in occupational therapy? For example, perhaps the client just underwent a strenuous medical treatment or just had physical therapy, which is the reason why the client is now tired, doesn't feel well, or performs poorly.

Morreale MJ, Borcherding S.
The OTA's Guide to Documentation:
Writing SOAP Notes, Third Edition (pp 99-112).
© 2013 SLACK Incorporated.

	Table 12-1 (continued)	
	Documenting Observations Accurately	
Client Factors, Performance Skills, and Environment	**"O"—What are your professional observations?** *Consider some of the following suggestions regarding your client that you might elaborate upon:*	**"A"—What professional words summarize your relevant observations for the assessment?** *You might choose from the following suggestions, then describe why that matters for your client:*
Affect/Demeanor and Behavior	• Client's stated mood? • Nonverbal communication? • Client's facial expression? • Client tearful/crying and for how long? • How is client consoled? • Posture? • Examples of defense mechanisms noted? • Energy or activity level? • What did client do and say? • Specific positive or negative statements made? • Expresses harmful thoughts regarding self or others? • What is client's stated opinion or outlook? • Response to intervention? • Task behaviors? • Approach to new or difficult situations? • Attention to detail? • Examples of problem-solving ability? • Expresses awareness of deficits? • Client's assessment of own abilities, appearance, etc? • Ability to overcome obstacles? • Ability to complete task? • Does client prefer to be alone or with others? • Kinds of relationships? • Many friends? • Interpersonal skills? • Specific decision-making skills observed? • Is encouragement needed? • Does client engage easily with others or in new situations? • Does client's behavior/speech make others uncomfortable or scared? • Does client use profane language, yell, or scream? • Does client express realistic or unrealistic fears/anxieties? • Does client exhibit negative behaviors such as hitting, kicking, spitting, or hurting others? • Frequency and duration of repetitive behaviors and rituals? • Client's stated attitude toward task completion? • Does client prefer structure or can "go with the flow?" • Does client express willingness to change thoughts or behavior? • Does client learn from mistakes? • Is client easily persuaded or will stick to an opinion or decision?	• Self-confidence • Self-esteem • Self-awareness • Decisiveness • Determination • Calmness • Enthusiasm • Trusting nature • Careful approach • Careless behavior • Resilience • Pessimistic outlook • Inconsolable • Grief-stricken mood • Suicidal ideation • Depressed mood • Expressive speech • Animated behavior • Outgoing personality • Sociable behavior • Cautious approach • Frustration tolerance • Attention to detail • Organizational skills • Flat affect • Shyness • Timidity • Withdrawn behavior • Passivity • Indecisiveness • Hesitancy regarding… • Vacillates… • Uncertainty regarding… • Flexibility • Rigidity • Anxiety/anxious behavior • Hyperactivity • Boredom • Indifference to… • Suspicious behavior • Risky behavior • Unsafe… • Carelessness when… • Easily distracted by… • Threatening speech/behavior • Aggressive behavior • Attentiveness • Patience • Optimistic outlook • Happy mood • Content • Unwavering • Perseveration • Motivation

(continued)

Table 12-1 (continued) Documenting Observations Accurately		
Client Factors, Performance Skills, and Environment	**"O"—What are your professional observations?** *Consider some of the following suggestions regarding your client that you might elaborate upon:*	**"A"—What professional words summarize your relevant observations for the assessment?** *You might choose from the following suggestions, then describe why that matters for your client:*
Motor Function	• Joint mobility and range? • Joint stability and alignment? • Does client have isolated, voluntary movement? • Quality and symmetry of movement noted? • Timing? • Are tremors evident at rest or upon AROM? • Are involuntary or excessive movements noted? • Are muscles well-defined? • Muscle grades? • End feels? • Excessive or abnormal tone evident? • Restrictions noted? • Is client at risk for falling? • Base of support? • Reciprocal motion? • Substitution or compensatory motions evident? • Do joints creak? • Is stretching needed to increase ROM? • Pain reported or not?	• Stable • Coordinated • Strong • Muscular • Atrophy • Powerful • Well-developed • Unrestricted • Flexible • Supple • Restricted motion • Agile • Limber • Volitional movement • Unsteady • Uncoordinated • Tremors • Ataxia • Rigidity • Flaccidity • Weak • Hypotonic • Subluxation • Stiffness • Tightness • Hypertonic • Hypermobility • Spasticity • Crepitation • Muscle twitching • Spasm
Physical Environment	• Type and level of dirt/grime? • Are items in proper place? • Can client locate items easily? • Noise level and types of auditory/visual distractions? • Specific fall hazards? • Sharps hazards? • Fire hazards? • Childproofing needed? • Presence/quantity of insects or rodents? • Mold present/amount? • Rotting food or open containers? • Raw sewage/pet waste? • Exposed electrical wires? • Garbage not in proper containers? • Areas inaccessible due to piles of… (e.g., clothes, garbage, food containers, boxes, etc.)? • Specific physical or architectural barriers?	• Organized • Neat • Clean • Unorganized • Messy • Cluttered • Unclean • Quiet environment • Noisy environment • Safe • Unsafe • Hazardous • Hoarding • Accessible • Inaccessible

(continued)

Table 12-1 (continued) ## Documenting Observations Accurately		
Client Factors, Performance Skills, and Environment	***"O"—What are your professional observations?*** *Consider some of the following suggestions regarding your client that you might elaborate upon:*	***"A"—What professional words summarize your relevant observations for the assessment?*** *You might choose from the following suggestions, then describe why that matters for your client:*
Communication/ Speech	• What is the client's native language? • Does the client speak English? • Is client able to speak, read, or write? • Is client willing to speak? • Can you hear what client is saying? • Can you understand what client is saying? • Can client modulate speech and tone of voice? • Quality of speech and flow? • Speech cadence? • Difficulty recalling words? • Does the client's speech make sense? • Does client understand what is said or written? • Can client answer questions, respond to commands, and express ideas effectively? • Is speech age-appropriate? • Is speech relevant to the situation? • Does client repeat things over and over? • Profanity or threatening words exhibited? • Length of responses? • Oral-motor weakness or difficulty forming words? • Pain or missing teeth? • Social interaction skills? • Response time? • Accuracy? • Is client to the point?	• Fluent • Halting • Lucid • Coherent • Clear • Direct • Succinct • Articulate • Well-spoken • Expressive • Incoherent • Unintelligible • Rambling • Lisp • Garbled • Illogical • Verbose • Reticent • Echolalia • Perseveration • Uncommunicative • Expressive aphasia • Receptive aphasia • Slurred speech • Dysphasia • Oral apraxia • Word-finding difficulties

Complete Worksheets 12-1 and 12-2 to review the mechanics of documentation and terminology that you learned in Chapters 2, 4, and 5. Then, complete Worksheets 12-3, 12-4, and 12-5 to help you integrate the suggestions in this chapter with information you learned in the previous chapters. The worksheets will help you to start making professional observations and use clinical reasoning skills for writing your own original SOAP notes. You may practice writing SOAP notes using Figure 12-1 on page 112 or Figure 2-1 in Chapter 2 of this book.

A Quick Checklist for Evaluating Your Note

Use the following two summary charts as a quick reference guide to ensure that your note contains all of the essential elements.

	S: Subjective	
☐	1.	Use something significant the client says about his treatment or condition.
	O: Objective	
☐	1.	Begin this section with:
☐		○ Indication of active client engagement/participation
☐		○ Length of session
☐		○ Setting
☐		○ Purpose of session
☐	2.	Report your observations succinctly and accurately, either chronologically or using categories.
☐	3.	Remember to do the following:
☐		○ De-emphasize the treatment media
☐		○ Specify what part of the task required assistance
☐		○ Specify the exact type and amount of assistance needed
☐		○ Use professional language and standard abbreviations
☐		○ Show skilled OT happening
☐		○ Leave yourself out
☐		○ Focus on the client's response
☐		○ Avoid being judgmental
	A: Assessment	
☐	1.	Look at the data in your "S" and "O" sentence by sentence, asking yourself what problems, progress, and rehab potential you see.
☐	2.	Ask yourself, "So what? Why is this important in the client's life?" For each underlying factor not within functional limits, identify the impact it will have on an area of occupation.
☐	3.	End the "A" with *"Client would benefit from..."*
☐		○ Justify continued skilled OT
☐		○ Set up the plan
☐	4.	Be sure the time lines and activities you are putting in your plan match the skilled OT you indicate your client needs.
	P: Plan	
☐	1.	Specify the frequency and duration of OT treatment.
☐	2.	Tell what you will be working on during that time to address the client's needs.
☐	3.	Relate to a performance skill/area of occupation and client's OT goals.
☐	4.	Indicate any other pertinent follow-up needed for the client's present situation.
	Remember to:	
☐		Include the client's identifying information, delineate OT department and type of note.
☐		Correct errors properly, do not erase or use correction fluid, and do not leave blank spaces.
☐		Make certain engagement in occupation is integral to the note.
☐		Sign and date your note.

Morreale, M. J., & Borcherding, S. (2013). *The OTA's guide to documentation: Writing SOAP notes (3rd ed.).* Thorofare, NJ: SLACK Incorporated.

S: Subjective
- ☐ Use something **significant** the client says about his **treatment** or **condition**.
- ☐ If there is nothing significant, ask yourself whether you are using your interview skills to elicit the proper information about how the client sees things.

O: Objective
- ☐ Begin this section with length of session, where the client was seen, and for what purpose. Make sure you indicate active client participation. For example,
    Client participated in 30-minute OT session in hospital room for instruction in compensatory dressing techniques.
- ☐ Summarize what you see, either chronologically or using categories.
- ☐ Focus on performance skills and de-emphasize the treatment media. For example,
    Client worked on three-point pinch using pegs.
- ☐ Relate preparatory activities and physical agent modalities to occupational performance.
    Client worked on three-point pinch using pegs in order to manage buttons on clothing.
- ☐ Specify the **part** of the task needing assistance and the exact **type** and **amount** of assistance provided.
    Client required five verbal cues for correct hand placement during w/c ↔ toilet transfers.
- ☐ Indicate that the client **needed** assistance rather than labeling the client as an assist level.
    "Client required min assist..." rather than *"Client is min assist..."*
- ☐ Use standardized terminology to grade and describe treatment interventions and client performance.
- ☐ Show skilled OT happening—make it clear that you were not just a passive observer. For example, do not just list all of the assist levels and think that is enough.
- ☐ Write from the client's point of view, leaving yourself out.
    "Client was repositioned in w/c..." rather than *"COTA repositioned client in w/c..."*
- ☐ Focus on the client's response rather than on what you did.
    Client able to don socks using sock aid after demonstration.
- ☐ Avoid judging the client. For example,
    Say client *"...didn't complete the activity."* Don't add *"...because he was stubborn."*

A: Assessment
- ☐ Look at the data in your "S" and "O" sentence by sentence, identifying problems, progress, and rehab potential. Ask yourself what each statement means for the client's occupational performance. Consider the following formula:

Underlying Limiting Factor	Functional Impact	Ability to Engage in Occupation

    For example, if in your "O" you noted that client falls to the left when sitting unsupported, what do you think this means he will be unable to do for himself? For example,
    Client unable to sit EOB unsupported to dress.
- ☐ Make sure you have not introduced any new information.
- ☐ End the "A" with *"Client would benefit from..."*
- ☐ Justify continued skilled OT.
    Client would benefit from skilled instruction in use of adaptive devices and compensatory techniques for performing IADL tasks one-handed.
- ☐ Set up the plan and match time lines in your plan to the skilled OT you document that your client needs. For example, if you justify skilled OT by saying only, *"Client would benefit from skilled instruction in energy conservation techniques,"* then do not say that you plan to treat client twice a day for 2 weeks. Skilled instruction in energy conservation should take only one session or, at most, two sessions.

P: Plan
- ☐ Specify the frequency, duration of treatment, and specific OT interventions that will be implemented.
- ☐ Identify the performance skills and the areas of occupation that will be addressed during that time.
    Continue OT 1 hour daily for 2 weeks for upper body strengthening and instruction in adaptive devices needed for safe and Ⓘ transfers to bed, toilet, and tub.

Morreale, M. J., & Borcherding, S. (2013). *The OTA's guide to documentation: Writing SOAP notes (3rd ed.).* Thorofare, NJ: SLACK Incorporated.

Worksheet 12-1
Mechanics of Documentation

Certain basic elements must be present in all documentation formats. Look at the following contact note and see how many elements you can find that are incorrect or missing. Realize that this note reflects a "special situation" and, therefore, does not need to include the complete S, O, A, and P format.

XYZ School District
Albany, NY

John Doe

3/22/12 Upon arrival to OT room, student reported he had a headache, felt nauseous, and stated he was "burning up." OT session defered and student escorted to ~~teach~~ nurse's office.

C. Caring, COTA

1.

2.

3.

4.

5.

6.

7.

8.

9.

10.

Morreale, M. J., & Borcherding, S. (2013). *The OTA's guide to documentation: Writing SOAP notes (3rd ed.)*. Thorofare, NJ: SLACK Incorporated.

Worksheet 12-2
Documentation Basics

For each of the following SOAP note sentences, correct any errors in spelling, grammar, abbreviations, and basic mechanics of documentation.

1. The client used compensitory techniques to donn his shoes and socks.

2. The client performed bed mobility Ⓘ, then sat on SOB with SBA to doff his shirt.

3. Child was seen for 20 minutes in classroom to help her put her coat on.

4. Client stated he will "not wear his splint to work."

5. The CVA pt. demonstrated ability to transfer bed ↔ commode with SBA and VC.

6. The child demonstrated progress by using her bad hand to stabilize the paper when writing.

7. During her Occupational Therapy session, the pt. worked on ↑ Ⓛ neglect and ↓ safety to perform ADLs.

8. I instructed the client in arom exercises to improve her ability to braid her two daughter's hair.

9. The client performed self-feeding with modified assistance.

10. The THR client's Ⓛ hip is sore because the PT made her walk too long.

11. The student was mod assist to write her name.

Morreale, M. J., & Borcherding, S. (2013). *The OTA's guide to documentation: Writing SOAP notes (3rd ed.)*. Thorofare, NJ: SLACK Incorporated.

Worksheet 12-3
Improving Observation Skills

Try an activity with a partner to improve your observation and documentation skills. Realize that this is simply a creative role-playing exercise.

Pretend your partner has had a stroke and cannot use the dominant upper extremity. Pick a BADL or IADL to work on (e.g., putting on a shoe or jacket, making a sandwich, etc.) and teach your partner compensatory techniques, just as you would a client. Now, using the suggestions in this chapter as a guide, list the following:

WHO

WHAT

WHERE

WHEN

WHY

HOW

Using this information, now write a SOAP note regarding your partner's "treatment session" on a separate page.

Morreale, M. J., & Borcherding, S. (2013). *The OTA's guide to documentation: Writing SOAP notes (3rd ed.).* Thorofare, NJ: SLACK Incorporated.

Worksheet 12-4
Improving Observation Skills—More Practice

Now try another activity with a partner to improve your observation and documentation skills. Realize that this is simply a creative role-playing exercise.

Pretend your partner has arthritis or COPD and has decreased upper extremity AROM and difficulty performing daily activities. Pick one BADL or IADL to work on (e.g., cooking, grooming, managing fastenings) and teach joint protection, energy conservation, or compensatory techniques. Also, teach your partner some exercises to improve AROM. Then, use the suggestions in this chapter to list the following:

WHO

WHAT

WHERE

WHEN

WHY

HOW

Using this information, now write a SOAP note regarding your partner's "treatment session" on a separate page.

Morreale, M. J., & Borcherding, S. (2013). *The OTA's guide to documentation: Writing SOAP notes (3rd ed.).* Thorofare, NJ: SLACK Incorporated.

Worksheet 12-5
Video Observation Skills

Using an Internet search engine, find a video of an OT treatment session or a video demonstrating use of an adaptive device or technique. Consider the suggestions in this chapter as you carefully watch and analyze the video. Write down your observations of the "client" and situation shown in the video. Realize this is simply a creative writing exercise to practice your observation skills.

WHO

WHAT

WHERE

WHEN

WHY

HOW

Using this information, write a SOAP note on a separate page regarding the "client" in the video.

Morreale, M. J., & Borcherding, S. (2013). *The OTA's guide to documentation: Writing SOAP notes (3rd ed.)*. Thorofare, NJ: SLACK Incorporated.

XYZ Home Health Care Agency
□ OT   □ PT   □ ST Department
Progress Note

Name: _____   Record #: _____

Dx: _____   SOC: _____

Date	

Figure 12-1. Example of a facility form.

Chapter 13

Making Good Notes Even Better

This chapter will help you review the four sections of the SOAP note. Complete the worksheets to practice what you have learned and to improve your skills.

Writing the "S"—Subjective

This section includes anything significant the client says regarding treatment. When you are working with a young child or a client who is confused or unable to communicate, you may report on nonverbal communication or state what the primary caregiver says. Sometimes inexperienced OTAs simply list anything important the client had to say about his condition, but that is not always appropriate. In Worksheet 13-2, all of the information is relevant, but does not form a coherent whole. It is better to condense and organize the information to make the "S" more concise.

Morreale MJ, Borcherding S.
The OTA's Guide to Documentation:
Writing SOAP Notes, Third Edition (pp 113-123).
© 2013 SLACK Incorporated.

Worksheet 13-1
SOAPing Your Note

Indicate which section of the SOAP note you would place each of the following statements.

1. ____ Client supine → sit in bed Ⓘ.

2. ____ Client moved kitchen items from counter to cabinet Ⓘ using Ⓛ hand.

3. ____ Parent reports child's handwriting has significantly improved within the past month.

4. ____ Problems include decreased coordination, strength, sensation, and proprioception in left hand, which create safety risks in home management tasks.

5. ____ Client reports that his fingers are stiff this morning and that he is having trouble handling small items like buttons.

6. ____ By the end of next treatment session, client will demonstrate ability to don/doff splint Ⓘ.

7. ____ Increase of 15 minutes in activity tolerance for UE activities permits her to prepare a light meal Ⓘ.

8. ____ Child participated in 30-minute OT session to promote development of FM skills for BADLs.

9. ____ Deficits in proprioception and motor planning limit client's ability to dress herself.

10. ____ Continue ROM and retrograde massage to Ⓡ hand for edema control and to enable grasp of objects needed for BADLs.

11. ____ Consumer will be seen 2X weekly to improve attention to task in order to obtain a job.

12. ____ Client reports that she cannot remember her hip precautions.

13. ____ Client would benefit from further instruction to incorporate total hip precautions into lower body dressing, bathing, and toilet hygiene.

14. ____ Learning was evident by client's ability to improve with repetition.

15. ____ Client's request to take rest breaks demonstrates knowledge of her limitations in endurance.

16. ____ Client required three verbal prompts to interact with peers in OT social group.

17. ____ Fair+ muscle grade of extension in Ⓡ wrist extensors this week shows good progress toward goals.

18. ____ Poor temporal organization interferes with getting to work on time.

19. ____ Next session, instruct parent in proper positioning of infant for bottle feeding.

20. ____ Client demonstrated ability to perform sliding board transfer w/c ↔ mat with min assist to position board properly.

Morreale, M. J., & Borcherding, S. (2013). *The OTA's guide to documentation: Writing SOAP notes (3rd ed.).* Thorofare, NJ: SLACK Incorporated.

Worksheet 13-2
Writing the "S"—Subjective

Try to write a more concise version of the following "S."

Client told OTA she has very bad arthritis in her Ⓡ shoulder and Ⓡ knee.
Client said, "It really hurts a lot to stand on my right leg."
Client described Ⓡ LE pain as 7/10 when weightbearing.
Client stated, "It [sliding board] needs to be moved further up on the seat."
When asked if she was ok after the transfer, client said, "I'm just tired."
Client stated, "I'm through," and requested help to get closer to the bed.
When client transferred to the bed, she said, "This is the hardest transfer for me."
Client stated she prefers to approach transfers from her Ⓡ side.

S:

Writing the "O"—Objective

Your observations are summarized and recorded in this section, either chronologically or in categories. Start with a statement indicating active client participation, where the client was seen, length of session, and purpose. The "O" focuses on the client's response to the intervention provided. Remember to de-emphasize the treatment media, and describe assist levels accurately. Try to show your professional skill in the first sentence but keep the focus on the client, not the OTA. Consider this example of a client whose limited mobility is compromising his positioning. Rather than saying, *"Client seen for positioning,"* a better choice of an opening sentence would be:

- *Client and spouse participated in 25-minute session in home for education on positioning to prevent skin breakdown.*
- *Client participated in 30-minute session in rehab gym for assessment of w/c positioning to improve sitting posture for mealtimes.*
- *Pt. participated in 40-minute session bedside for positioning strategies to minimize risk of falling out of w/c.*

Complete Worksheet 13-3 to practice writing good opening lines in the "O" part of the note.

Morreale, M. J., & Borcherding, S. (2013). *The OTA's guide to documentation: Writing SOAP notes (3rd ed.).* Thorofare, NJ: SLACK Incorporated.

Worksheet 13-3
Making Opening Lines Better

Rewrite the following opening sentences to show how your skill as an OTA is important in each situation.

1. **Old opening sentence**: *Client practiced laundry tasks for 45 minutes.*
   Additional information:
   - Client has total hip precautions, which raise safety concerns during functional mobility, especially during performance of household chores.
   - Adaptive equipment is available if needed.

2. **Old opening sentence**: *Consumer seen at workshop for 1 hour to improve job skills.*
   Additional information:
   - Deficits in time management skills ↓ his ability to work Ⓘ.
   - Bilateral coordination problems interfere with client completing an essential job function of opening/closing boxes.
   - ↓ tolerance to auditory stimuli contribute to client's high distractibility during task completion.

3. **Old opening sentence**: *Client seen in his hospital room bedside for 30 minutes for feeding.*
   Additional information:
   - Client has Ⓛ neglect.
   - Client's dominant hand is flaccid.
   - Adaptive equipment is available.

4. **Old opening sentence**: *Worked with client in kitchen for 1 hr. to ↑ Ⓘ in cooking.*
   Additional information:
   - Client's problems include decreased tolerance for standing and inattention of affected UE, which raise safety concerns.

Morreale, M. J., & Borcherding, S. (2013). *The OTA's guide to documentation: Writing SOAP notes (3rd ed.).* Thorofare, NJ: SLACK Incorporated.

Be Specific About Assist Levels

Remember that in addition to reporting the level of assistance needed, you also must be specific about the **part of the task** that required assistance.

Not specific enough:

Resident supine → sit with max Ⓐ, sit → stand mod Ⓐ.

Specific:

Resident supine → sit with max Ⓐ to lift legs over EOB, sit → stand with mod Ⓐ for balance and to maintain toe-touch weightbearing precautions with use of walker.

There is a difference between telling **why** the assist was needed, for example:

Client needed mod verbal cues to eat lunch due to perceptual deficits.

and **the part of the task** that required assistance:

Client needed mod verbal cues to locate utensils and food on Ⓛ side of meal tray.

It is helpful to list both the part of the task that needed assistance and the observable reason for why the assist was needed:

Client needed mod verbal cues to locate utensils and food on Ⓛ side of meal tray due to unilateral inattention.

Due to Ⓛ neglect, mod verbal cues were needed for client to locate all items on Ⓛ side of meal tray.

Make the "O" Complete and Concise

In the objective section of your note, you record your observations of the intervention session concisely. As you become more proficient, it becomes easier to determine what to include and what to omit. Below is an observation of a treatment session that is very concise.

Client was seen in hospital room for further ADL training. Client participated in BADLs and transfer activities.
BADLs
Client donned robe Ⓘ with set up.
Client donned/doffed socks Ⓘ with set-up.
Mobility
Bed → chair with CGA
Supine → sit Ⓘ

What problems are evident with this "O"?

This note is TOO concise and omits pertinent information. It lacks an indication that skilled occupational therapy was provided. This note could begin with an opening sentence that shows why your skill as an OTA is needed in this situation. As it stands, it is apparent that someone observed the client dress and transfer and recorded assist levels, but nursing staff or a rehabilitation aide could simply have done this.

Secondly, the activities documented in this note do not appear to require much time, so the session could be very short. If this is an hour treatment session, was anything else done? Was education or special instruction provided? If the client was slow to do the things recorded above, what caused so few activities to take such a long time? Is there a cognitive or perceptual problem? Is there a problem with coordination, safety, or motor planning? Did the client use compensatory techniques or adaptive equipment to be independent?

Third, as this note indicates the client is independent, there is nothing else in this note to justify that additional occupational therapy is necessary. Unless this is the final treatment session, there needs to be information provided that will justify continued treatment.

Worksheet 13-4
Writing the "O"—Objective

Now it is your turn to practice. Read the observation below and consider what this note needs to make it better. Instead of rewriting the entire note, just write suggestions to improve the note in the box below:

Toilet transfers: *mod Ⓐ*
Toileting: *min Ⓐ with SBA 2° inability to support self with Ⓛ arm and to dress*
UE dressing: *min Ⓐ, verbal cues, set up, Ⓘ in pulling shirt over head*
LE dressing: *used dressing stick*
        min Ⓐ pants to hips
        max Ⓐ pants to waist
        modified Ⓘ to don Ⓛ shoe (elastic shoelaces)
        modified Ⓘ to don Ⓡ shoe (elastic shoelaces)
Ⓡ hand status: *Ⓡ fingers: small has spasticity (index finger greatest amount)*
        Thumb: CMC joint painful in abduction
        Ⓡ wrist: flaccid

Suggestions to improve this note:

1.

2.

3.

4.

5.

Morreale, M. J., & Borcherding, S. (2013). *The OTA's guide to documentation: Writing SOAP notes (3rd ed.).* Thorofare, NJ: SLACK Incorporated.

Writing Effective Assessment Statements

It is sometimes difficult for a student or novice OTA to differentiate an observation from an assessment. An observation is anything you see a client **do** while your assessment is how it **impacts** an area of occupation. The assessment is your professional opinion about the meaning of what you have just observed in the intervention session. As you analyze the information you gathered, you will look for evidence of problems, progress (or lack of progress), and rehab potential. Problems may include any aspect of the occupational therapy domain that is not within functional limits or creates a concern (Gateley & Borcherding, 2012). The assessment is not the place to include any new information and it should end with a statement of what the client would benefit from. For example, for a client who has hip precautions and for whom you have observed some problem areas, you might say:

A: *Client's inability to remember hip precautions without verbal cues during IADLs puts her at risk for reinjury. Supportive daughter and ability to use adaptive equipment properly after instruction indicate a good potential for reaching stated goals. Client would benefit from further skilled instruction in maintaining hip precautions during IADL tasks, sit ↔ stand, and transitional living skills.*

You have learned a useful formula to assess the underlying factors that are not within functional limits. While not the only correct way to write assessments, this formula will help you to include all of the necessary components in your assessment.

Underlying Limiting Factor	Functional Impact	Ability to Engage in Occupation

There are several steps needed to assess an underlying factor that is not within functional limits:

- First determine what the basic deficit or problem is (such as *poor muscle strength, inability to attend to task, an environmental barrier,* or *a challenging aspect of the activity*).
- Make the problem or deficit the subject of your statement for emphasis.
- Determine whether the area of difficulty you have observed today is an indicator of a broader area of occupation. For example, is the decreased strength you observed causing a problem in grooming also creating problems in other basic ADL tasks? Will the client's depressed mood or poor attention cause difficulty with work tasks? Will the problems you observed today create any safety concerns or affect the ability to return home?
- Your assessment statement must relate how the problem areas impact the client's ability to engage in meaningful occupation. After each problem you note (e.g., limited strength, poor attention, depressed mood), ask yourself "So what?" So the client is unable to do that—how does this impact his or her life? The answer to your "So what" question becomes your assessment of the situation.
- Relate how the client would benefit from further occupational therapy. If no further occupational therapy is warranted or other recommendations are appropriate at this time, indicate why.

Let us now compare some observation and assessment statements.

Suppose you are working with a client who plans to return home to live alone in her apartment. Your intervention has included teaching her hip precautions following her total hip replacement, but she forgets to incorporate these when practicing home management tasks. What is this client's basic or core problem? Why does it matter or why is it important?

The following statement is an objective **observation** of the client's behavior:

Pt. was unable to adhere to hip precautions during laundry task due to memory deficit.

However, when phrased differently, it demonstrates the OTA's clinical reasoning and becomes an **assessment** of what was observed:

Memory deficit interferes with client's ability to adhere to total hip precautions, which limits her ability to safely perform self-care and IADL tasks needed to return to prior Ⓘ living situation.

The OTA has determined in the assessment that this client's basic problem is the inability to retain instructions. The OTA should then address this problem with a recommendation to use compensatory techniques (memory cues) of some kind. The safety concerns that impact the client's ability to return home should be considered. Otherwise, why should a third-party payer continue to pay for instruction that will not be remembered? According to the formula, rather than repeat what was observed, the assessment begins with the underlying problem, expands the scope of the area of occupation to include related tasks, (in this case IADLs and self-care tasks), and answers the question, "So what? Why does this matter in this client's life or why is it important?"

Sweeping Assessment Statements

Due to a busy schedule and time constraints, it can be tempting for an OTA to make brief and sweeping assessment statements such as:

A: *Deficits in upper body strength, fine motor skills, and feeding limit Jordan's ability to be Ⓘ in home and classroom activities.*

Although accurate, this statement is limited and would benefit from some elaboration. A better way to assess Jordan's information would be to say:

A: *Deficits in upper body strength limit Jordan's Ⓘ in eating, functional mobility, and dressing. Decreased fine motor skills impede typical classroom activities such as holding a pencil or crayon or manipulating small items, as well as age-appropriate IADL tasks in which Jordan is beginning to show an emerging interest. Jordan would benefit from continued upper body strengthening, reach-grasp-release tasks, and skilled feeding activities to move Jordan more expediently through typical developmental milestones.*

The assessment demonstrates your clinical reasoning as an OTA and enables others reading your note to better understand the client's situation.

Worksheet 13-5
Differentiating Between Observations and Assessments

Identify which of the statements below are observations and which are assessments.

1. ___ Client is unable to don Ⓛ LE prosthesis for functional mobility.

2. ___ Inability to don Ⓛ LE prosthesis Ⓘ prevents client from performing safe functional mobility around the house to live alone.

3. ___ Decreased tolerance to auditory stimuli limits the student's ability to attend to classroom tasks.

4. ___ Student required three verbal cues to stay on task due to decreased tolerance to auditory stimuli.

5. ___ Client was unable to incorporate relaxation and stress reduction techniques, requiring several verbal prompts to complete task.

6. ___ Inability to incorporate relaxation and stress reduction techniques when interacting with sales clerk limits her ability to manage shopping tasks Ⓘ after discharge.

Reword the following observations to make them **assessments**.

1. Client demonstrated difficulty with balancing checkbook due to memory and sequencing deficits.

2. Client unable to complete homemaking tasks or basic self-care activities independently due to Ⓛ neglect, impulsive behavior, and decreased attention to task.

3. After the use of behavior modification techniques, child demonstrated ability to remain seated at his desk for the remainder of the treatment session.

Worksheet 13-6
Problems, Progress, and Rehab Potential

For the following observation, note the problems or underlying factors not within functional limits. Then, list the information that indicates potential for progress.

O: *Client participated in 30-minute session in OT clinic to work on improving functional movements of ®️ UE, dynamic sitting balance, and cognitive skills. Client needed mod Ⓐ in shifting weight to get to edge of w/c and max verbal cues to use correct posture and shift feet during standing pivot transfer w/c → mat. Client required max verbal cues to initiate grasp of bag in beanbag activity. Client required mod Ⓐ to initiate reaching with ®️ UE but demonstrated ability to complete ®️ UE shoulder flexion required to toss bag appropriately 2 feet with max verbal cues. Client demonstrated cognitive understanding of activity with mod verbal cues by stating desired goal to be achieved by accurate aim.*

Problems:

Progress/Rehab Potential:

Assessment: How do the problems and progress you noted impact the client's ability to engage in meaningful occupation (such as safety concerns or ability to care for self)? What would the client benefit from? What skilled OT intervention is indicated? Integrate this information to write the "A" part of this note.

A.

Plan: Your plan contains a statement of how often and for how long you will be seeing the client and your treatment priorities toward the client's goals. For example:

P: *Continue OT 3 x wk for 1 wk to work on incorporating hip precautions into ADL tasks.*

While this plan states what intervention is necessary, it is not very specific. The plan should reflect your clinical reasoning and clarify what specific ADL or problem is a priority to address with the client.

P: *Continue OT 3 x wk for 1 wk to work on incorporating hip precautions into ADL tasks. Next session, instruct client in use of adaptive equipment for lower body dressing.*

Now finish the note with the plan.

P.

Morreale, M. J., & Borcherding, S. (2013). *The OTA's guide to documentation: Writing SOAP notes (3rd ed.).* Thorofare, NJ: SLACK Incorporated.

Worksheet 13-7
The "Almost" Note

Now it is your turn to integrate all you have learned. This note is **almost** good enough. In fact, it appears to be quite good on the surface, but actually has major flaws in organization and clinical reasoning. Mrs. M. is a 78-year-old female who sustained a Ⓛ CVA and has Ⓡ hemiparesis. Her OTA wrote the treatment note below. How can this note be improved? There is no need to try to rewrite the entire note. For this worksheet, simply make suggestions about what this note needs to be more effective.

S: *Client reports stiffness in Ⓡ hip, but improvement from previous pain. She states a preference for transferring to her left. Client states that she is willing to do "whatever it takes to get out of the hospital."*

O: *Client seen in room to work on dressing and functional mobility.*

Transfer: *Client SBA for standing pivot transfer bed → w/c to the left*
Client min Ⓐ with transfers w/c → toilet using grab bar

Mobility: *Client SBA with VCs to flex trunk when rolling from supine to Ⓡ side*
Client SBA supine → sit; min Ⓐ sit → stand
Client Ⓘ in w/c mobility

Dressing: *Client Ⓘ in donning shirt*
Client min Ⓐ with VCs to don bra while standing
Client Ⓘ in donning socks and shoes
Client min Ⓐ with walker and VCs in donning underwear and pants
Client needs setup for dressing activities

UE ROM: *Ⓛ UE—WFL*
Ⓡ UE—↓ range in shoulder flexion

Static standing: *Client SBA with walker*
Dynamic standing: *Client SBA with walker for balance*

A. *Deficits noted in Ⓡ UE coordination, Ⓑ UE strength, and dynamic standing balance. Client Ⓘ in dressing EOB, but is min Ⓐ in dressing when standing with a walker. Ⓛ UE AROM is WFL, but Ⓡ UE has deficits noted in shoulder flexion. Client needs SBA in bed mobility when rolling to unaffected side and min Ⓐ in sit → stand 2° ↓ UE strength. Client needs SBA for transfer to unaffected side in pivot transfer bed → w/c and min Ⓐ w/c → toilet. Client would benefit from skilled OT to continue UE strengthening and coordination exercises and to ↑ dynamic standing balance using walker in order to ↑ Ⓘ in ADLs.*

P: *Client to be seen twice daily for 30-minute sessions to continue to work on dynamic standing balance.*

Suggestions for improving the Almost Note:

Morreale, M. J., & Borcherding, S. (2013). *The OTA's guide to documentation: Writing SOAP notes (3rd ed.).* Thorofare, NJ: SLACK Incorporated.

Chapter 14

Evaluation and Intervention Planning

Referral Process

As discussed in Chapter 1, occupational therapy practitioners write different kinds of notes for different stages of the intervention process. The process begins when a client is referred to occupational therapy. In medical settings, this referral might also be called _doctor's orders, medical orders, prescription_, or _script_. The OT is responsible for responding to the new referral (AOTA, 2010c). It is important to realize that occupational therapy practice acts (licensure) may differ in key aspects from state to state. For example, practice acts delineate whether a prescription is required for evaluation and/or treatment and specify which health care professionals can legally write a referral for occupational therapy in that state (such as a physician, optometrist, nurse practitioner, or physician's assistant). States may also differ regarding continuing competency requirements or scope of practice, which delineates what the occupational therapy practitioner legally is allowed to do or may be prohibited from doing in that particular state (e.g., physical agent modalities). Each facility will have specific policies and procedures in place to facilitate the referral process according to the type of practice setting, licensure laws, and other ethical and legal requirements. Let us consider some examples of the referral process.

Inpatient Setting

For an inpatient setting such as a hospital or long-term care facility, a referral for occupational therapy is typically established in the health record by the physician (or other appropriate professional). Depending on the facility, this entry might be handwritten, entered by computer, faxed, or established as a verbal telephone order or other means. The occupational therapy referral could be initiated when the client is first admitted or might be established later as the need for occupational therapy arises. The occupational therapy department is then notified of the order by procedures established by the facility such as a computerized list, e-mail, or a call from the unit secretary. The client is then seen by the OT as soon as possible according to established guidelines.

Outpatient Setting

In an outpatient setting, when a new client calls, e-mails, or stops by to schedule an appointment, the occupational therapy department will consider the urgency of the appointment (such as if the patient must be seen that same day) and schedule it according to the client's needs and OT's schedule. The client's diagnosis, referral information, insurance, and contact information is usually verified during that initial contact.

Morreale MJ, Borcherding S.
The OTA's Guide to Documentation:
Writing SOAP Notes, Third Edition (pp 125-139).
© 2013 SLACK Incorporated.

School-Based Setting

In a school-based setting, the request for special services or occupational therapy might be initiated by a parent, teacher, or other staff. The request is considered by the Child Study Team and the child is evaluated as appropriate by the necessary disciplines. An Individualized Education Program (IEP) is then established to determine what specific services will be provided.

We will now look at each step of the occupational therapy evaluation process.

Overview

Very early in the process, an **intake note** may be written by the OT acknowledging the referral and stating a plan to evaluate. Next, the OT writes a screening or **evaluation report** that contains the client's occupational profile, current concerns and priorities, as well as the assessment results. From this comes the **intervention plan**, technically the part of the evaluation report that outlines the specific areas of occupation to be addressed, the outcomes expected, and the particular services that will be provided in occupational therapy. An OTA can contribute to this screening and evaluation process by performing delegated assessments and providing feedback and documentation to the OT (AOTA, 2010c). Facilities vary in the type, format, and frequency of **contact** or **progress notes** required. Some settings require a **contact note** (also called a *treatment note* or *visit note*) for each visit. Others may require a progress note every week, 2 weeks, 30 days, or more frequently for new referrals or for a change in status. Contact notes and progress notes are written by the OT or OTA (under the supervision of the OT) and often use the SOAP format you have learned in this manual. The requirements for type and frequency of notes are usually a function of the practice setting, payment source, and the accrediting agency. Sometimes a **reassessment note** is required at regular intervals. When a client is transferred from one setting to another within the same service delivery system, a **transition plan** may be written. Most facilities require a **discharge** or **discontinuation report** at the end of occupational therapy treatment. This report makes recommendations, summarizes the occupational therapy services provided, and notes changes in a client's ability to engage in meaningful occupation as a result of occupational therapy intervention. Reevaluation, transition, and discharge or discontinuation reports are the responsibility of the OT. However, the OTA may contribute to these stages of treatment by performing delegated assessments and providing feedback and documentation to the OT (AOTA, 2010c).

In actual practice, you will probably find that contact, progress, and reassessment notes have some overlap. For example, in outpatient settings, the contact notes often include the client's progress from session to session. Contact notes in practice settings where the client's status may change quickly, such as acute care, may seem much like progress notes. In some ways, progress notes reassess the client's status and may sound much like reassessment notes. Notes may also be named differently or combined in some service delivery systems. However, there are established basic guidelines for each kind of note.

Take another look at Chapter 2 to review the basics of documentation (such as client and facility identifying information, standards of signature, correcting errors, etc.). It would also be useful to review the description of skilled and unskilled services in Chapter 3. These criteria are applicable to all types of occupational therapy notes.

In *Guidelines for Documentation of Occupational Therapy* (AOTA, 2008a), criteria for notes in three process areas are described: evaluation, intervention, and outcome. Evaluation and screening reports, along with reassessment reports, are considered **evaluations**. The **intervention process** consists of the intervention plan, contact notes, progress reports, and transition plans. Discontinuation or discharge notes record professional activity in the area of **outcomes**. Occupational therapy practitioners must meet the often difficult challenge of providing complete, comprehensive, quality care and professional documentation within the time constraints often faced due to managed care. We will now look at documentation for evaluation and intervention planning.

Initial Evaluation Reports

The Evaluation Process

From the moment the referral is received, intervention planning begins in the mind of the OT. The client's name, age, and reason for referral will stimulate a good OT to begin reviewing in his or her mind the areas of occupation needing assessment, the areas of deficits likely to be found, and the possible interventions the OT might want to use.

Each client is different, of course, and there will be many variations, as well as some surprises as the assessment begins. The mental preparation for *"Andrew Smith, age 68, Ⓛ CVA, evaluate and treat"* takes a therapist on a mental journey along one road of thought, whereas *"Carrie Steed, age 4, ADHD,"* takes the therapist mentally down a different pathway. From day one, a good practitioner also begins discharge planning based on the client's occupational profile, prior functional level, and probable discharge placement.

In a medical or school setting, one of the first steps is a review of the client's record. This allows the OT to better understand the client's condition, determine the direction of the interview, and decide what assessments to administer. Information obtained from the health record might include the following:

- Primary and secondary diagnoses/reason for admission/hospitalization
- Medical orders—in addition to actual orders for therapy, these might include pertinent issues such as weightbearing status, type of diet (e.g., pureed, clear liquid, NPO, low salt), orthopedic or cardiac precautions, oxygen or MET levels, permission to get out of bed, etc.
- Medications
- Procedures or surgery implemented or pending
- Past medical history
- Test results such as X-rays, lab tests, MRIs, or neurological, developmental, or psychological tests
- Living situation and expected discharge plan
- Information from other disciplines such as physical or speech therapy evaluation results and goals

Data are also obtained from the client, family/caregiver, and other pertinent sources. Sometimes it is necessary for occupational therapy practitioners to talk to the nursing staff or contact the physician directly to clarify orders or discuss the client's condition or precautions before the client is seen. In early intervention and school settings, the therapist will review the child's available information and collaborate as needed with the parents, teachers, and other appropriate disciplines, such as social work, speech therapy, or psychology. The OT determines what information is needed for the client's occupational profile. This includes focusing on the client's occupational history, determining what that client needs and wants from occupational therapy, as well as what factors impact engagement in occupation. The OT selects and administers any standardized tests or survey instruments that will help determine more exactly what underlying factors support or hinder participation in occupations. The therapist might delegate some aspects of the chart review, interview, specific assessments, or other functions to the OTA.

If the client is verbal and oriented, an interview is top on the agenda. If the client is unable to provide information, the family or other caregiver may be able to provide the necessary information instead. The occupational therapy practitioner must ask questions to determine the client's occupational profile and find out what roles are important to this client. What areas of life present the most problems? What does the client hope to gain from treatment? What results are desired by the family or teacher? What was the client able to do prior to this injury, illness, or hospitalization? What supports are available to facilitate the desired outcomes? Often, much information is gleaned from simply watching the client enter into the treatment area, classroom, or other venue. Does the client guard for pain? Is a supportive family member accompanying the client? What is the quality of mobility, posture, and upper extremity motion or function that is evident? Are there apparent cognitive or perceptual problems? Are there obvious social, behavioral, or interpersonal concerns? Formal and informal assessments will then be administered based on the client's condition and practice setting and influenced by what third-party payers are looking for. These might include instruments relating to areas of occupation such as the Canadian Occupational Performance Measure (COPM); Functional Independence Measure (FIM); a leisure inventory; functional observations (e.g., ADLs, play, classroom performance); or various standardized or informal cognitive, perceptual, motor, sensory, developmental, or other tests to assess specific performance skills or client factors.

Considering the initial evaluation findings, the OT will identify and prioritize the areas of occupation and underlying factors that require attention, and develop an intervention plan. Most facilities provide forms for an initial evaluation report. The assessment results are recorded on the form, along with pertinent observations and comments. Some specific assessments might be recorded on a separate form designated for that particular test (e.g., goniometry, manual muscle testing) but are still included as part of the evaluation report. Facilities sometimes use the same form for reevaluation and discharge reports so that the evaluation material does not have to be rewritten. An example of an initial evaluation form from Capitol Region Medical Center in Jefferson City, MO (Figure 14-1) is presented in this chapter so that you can see what might be included on a good facility form. Note that this form emphasizes some areas of occupation (ADLs) over others (such as social participation or play) based on the type of practice setting. You can use an Internet search engine to find other examples of forms and compare different formats.

CAPITAL REGION MEDICAL CENTER
OCCUPATIONAL THERAPY
☐ **INITIAL EVALUATION** ☐ **DISCHARGE SUMMARY**

DIAGNOSIS _____ONSET: _____

_____

MED. HX: _____

_____CODE STATUS: _____

RELEVANT SURG. PROC.:_____

REFERRAL DATE: _____DATE: _____

REFERRING PHYSICIAN:_____MEDICARE #: _____

ACTIVITIES OF DAILY LIVING   REHAB POTENTIAL:_____

DRESSING Put on & remove the following	INDEP	SBA	MIN. ASSIST	MOD. ASSIST	MAX. ASSIST	ADAPT. EQUIP.	COMMENTS/ADAPTIVE EQUIPMENT ISSUED
front opening shirt							
pull on shirt							
underwear							
bra							
pants/slacks							
socks/hose							
shoes							
manage fasteners							
braces/splints/prosthesis							
GROOMING/HYGIENE							
sponge bath							
tub/shower bath							
shave							
comb hair							
brushing teeth							
opens jars/bottles							
make-up							
EATING							
drink from cup/glass							
feeds self							
cuts meat							

ROM — **UPPER EXTREMITY ROM & STRENGTH**

ACTIVE LEFT	PASSIVE LEFT	ACTIVE RIGHT	PASSIVE RIGHT		STRENGTH L	R
				SHOULDER: Elevation		
				Flexion		
				Abduction		
				Horizontal Abduction		
				Horizontal Adduction		
				Internal Rotation		
				External Rotation		
				ELBOW: Flexion		
				Extension		
				Supination		
				Pronation		
				WRIST: Flexion		
				Shoulder Subluxation L R		
				UE Edema L R		
				Pain L R		

PERTINENT FINDINGS

Wears glasses_____ Dentures_____ Hearing_____

MUSCLE TONE/UPPER EXTREMITIES

Hypotonic_____ Normal_____ Hypertonic_____
Comments_____

UPPER EXTREMITY SENSATION

SENSATION	Intact	Impaired	Absent
Light touch			
Sharp/Dull			
Temperature			
Proprioception			
Stereognosis			

COORDINATION/UPPER EXTREMITIES

Tremors_____ Apraxia_____ Ataxic_____

	Impaired	WNL
Gross Motor		
Fine Motor		
9 Hole Peg Test	L	R
Grip Strength	L	R
Lateral Pinch	L	R
Tripod Pinch	L	R
Hand Dominance	L	R

ORIENTED TO:

Person_____ Place_____
Time: Month_____ Day_____ Year_____
Situation_____

COMMUNICATION/COGNITION

	YES	NO
Verbal		
Understandable		
Appropriate		
Perseveration		
Follows Simple Commands		
Reads		
Writes		

2,605,003 (9/99) INIT. EVAL./DISCHG. SUM. (FRONT)

PERCEPTION

A.   R/L Neglect_____

	Impaired	WNL
B. Body Schema		
C. Discrimination		
Shape		
Size		
Color		
D. Visual Perception		

Overall Endurance   WFL_____
Fair_____
Poor_____

SURVIVAL SKILLS	Indep.	Min. Assist	Mod. Assist	Max. Assist
Phone Book Usage				
Money Mngmt.				
Situational Problem Solving				
Homemaking				

Figure 14-1A. Occupational therapy initial evaluation and discharge report form (page 1). (Reprinted with permission of Capital Region Medical Center, Jefferson City, MO.)

HOME SITUATION:_____

LIVING ARRANGEMENTS: (PT ADDRESS) _____

HOME TYPE:_____

PRIOR FUNCTIONAL INDEP.:_____

_____

_____

LEISURE INTERESTS:_____

ADAPTIVE EQUIP.:_____

COMMENTS:_____

_____

_____

_____

PATIENT / FAMILY GOALS:_____

❏ INITIAL ASSESSMENT (PROBLEMS / STRENGTHS)   ❏ DISCHARGE STATUS OF SHORT / LONG TERM GOALS

_____

_____

_____

_____

_____

PLAN:_____

SHORT-TERM GOALS - ESTIMATED TIME TO ACHIEVE: _____

_____

_____

_____

_____

❏ LONG-TERM GOALS - ESTIMATED TIME TO ACHIEVE: ❏ RECOMMENDATIONS:

_____

_____

_____

_____

_____

❏ Yes   ❏ No   **Patient has participated in evaluation process and agrees with treatment plan as stated above.**

Therapist _____   Date_____

I have reviewed and agree with the treatment plan as stated above.

Physician Signature _____   Date_____

2,605,003 (9/99) OT INITIAL EVALUATION/DISCHARGE SUMMARY (BACK)

Figure 14-1B. Occupational therapy initial evaluation and discharge report form (page 2). (Reprinted with permission of Capital Region Medical Center, Jefferson City, MO.)

If an initial evaluation is written as a SOAP note, this is the way information would be categorized.
   S: The interview material, background information, and occupational profile
   O: The tests, results, and clinical observations
   A: The OT's professional assessment of the data presented in the S and the O (often written as a problem list)
   P: Frequency and duration of planned interventions and the long- and short-term goals
You will find that facilities vary in how they organize and present the information. Forms may include checklists, grids, fill in the blanks, or spaces for narrative reports. Several different formats are used in this manual to make it clear that there is not one correct organizational strategy.

The *Guidelines for Documentation of Occupational Therapy* (AOTA, 2008a) recommend the following criteria for the content of an evaluation or screening report:

---

1.   Documents the referral source and data gathered through the evaluation process, including
   a.   Description of the client's occupational profile
   b.   Analysis of occupational performance and identification of factors that hinder and support performance in areas of occupation
   c.   Delineation of specific areas of occupation and occupational performance that will be targeted for intervention and outcomes expected.

2.   An abbreviated evaluation process (e.g., screening) documents only limited areas of occupation and occupational performance applicable to the client and to the situation.

3.   Suggested content with examples includes
   a.   *Client information*—name/agency, date of birth, gender, health status, applicable medical/educational/developmental diagnoses, precautions, and contraindications
   b.   *Referral information*—date and source of referral, services requested, reason for referral, funding source, and anticipated length of service
   c.   *Occupational profile*—client's reason for seeking occupational therapy services, current areas of occupation that are successful and problematic, contexts and environments that support and hinder occupations, medical/educational/work history, occupational history (e.g., patterns of living, interest, values), client's priorities, and targeted outcomes
   d.   *Assessments used and results*—types of assessments used and results (e.g., interviews, record reviews, observations, standardized or nonstandardized assessments), and confidence in test results
   e.   *Analysis of occupational performance*—description of and judgment about performance skills, performance patterns, contexts and environments, features of the activities, and client factors that facilitate and inhibit performance
   f.   *Summary and analysis*—interpretation and summary of data as it is related to occupational profile and referring concern
   g.   *Recommendation*—judgment regarding appropriateness of occupational therapy services or other services.

   Note: Intervention goals addressing anticipated outcomes, objectives, and frequency of therapy are listed on the Intervention Plan.

Reprinted with permission from American Occupational Therapy Association. (2008a). Guidelines for documentation of occupational therapy. *American Journal of Occupational Therapy, 62*(6), 684–690.

In an evaluation, the "S" may contain all or part of the occupational profile. Based on the above guidelines, some specific areas to consider might be:
- The client's living situation—type of dwelling, architectural barriers, who resides with the client, access to family or community services
- Client's responsibility for caring for children, pets, or others
- Roles, responsibilities, and ability to care for self
- Performance patterns—typical day, limiting behaviors
- Cultural and spiritual considerations—dietary or religious issues, personal values, customs

- Educational considerations—level of education, literacy, special skills, goals
- Occupation—paid or volunteer work, is client working now, did injury occur on the job, desire to return to work, work capabilities
- Play/leisure—opportunity and barriers regarding leisure, hobbies/interests, sedentary versus active leisure tasks
- Community mobility—methods of transportation, barriers to mobility
- Community support systems
- Virtual—access, competency, barriers
- Social—type and level of participation, clubs/organizations, successful relationships, opportunities and barriers
  Here are two examples of the "S" in a paragraph format.

> *Client reports that she was admitted after a fall that resulted in confusion and left-sided weakness. Prior to admission, she was living alone in a one-story home and was Ⓘ in all activities of daily living. She reports that she is a retired librarian, widowed 10 years ago. Client states she values her independence and fully intends to return to her own home. She reports that her activities are primarily sedentary, including sewing, reading, and playing cards with friends. She states her daughter lives two blocks away and provides transportation when needed.*

> *The client talked about his current symptoms and the events leading up to his hospitalization. He reports losing his job with a construction company after not reporting for work for 2 weeks due to depression, having an argument with his wife, and taking an overdose. He states that he has always "worked construction" and does not know how to do anything else. He reports concern that his former employer will not give him "a decent reference." He expresses he really has no leisure interests except going out "drinking with the guys after work" and sometimes going hunting in the fall.*

Review the following example of an initial evaluation report and intervention plan. Note that the occupational profile contained in this note is organized into categories rather than written as a paragraph.

Healthy Hospital
Occupational Therapy Department
Initial Evaluation Report

Name: Payshent, Polly   **Medical Record #**: 12345   **Insurance**: Medicare
DOB: 11/10/1943   **Age**: 68   **Sex**: F
Physician: Will Heelue, MD
Date of onset: 5/1/12   **Date of admission**: 5/2/12
Referral Data: Client referred 5/3/12 by Dr. Heelue for evaluation and treatment.
Primary Dx: Ⓡ CVA r/o OBS   **Secondary Dx**: Type 2 diabetes
Date of evaluation: 5/3/12   **Time**: 10:00 am
Occupational Profile:
  History of present condition: Client was admitted from the ER after a fall at home on 5/1/2012, resulting in confusion and left-sided weakness. CT scan and MRI both positive for Ⓡ CVA.
  Prior level of function: Prior to admission, client was Ⓘ in all activities of daily living.
  Living situation: Client lives alone in a one-story home with 3 steps to enter. Spouse deceased 10 years. Daughter works for United Wickets, lives 2 blocks away, and is willing to visit daily and assist with transportation but cannot provide supervision.
  Work: Client is a retired librarian.
  Social/Leisure: Hobbies include mostly sedentary activities such as sewing, reading, and playing cards with friends.
  Client's goals: Client states she values her independence and fully intends to return to her own home.
  S: Client stated, "I'm doing this so I can be independent and go home."
  O: Client participated in OT session bedside and in shower room for Mini-Mental State Exam, evaluation of personal ADL tasks (toileting, dressing ↔ undressing, and showering) functional mobility, and underlying factors (manual muscle test, AROM)
       Bathing: Upper body: min Ⓐ to sequence task; Lower body: min Ⓐ except max Ⓐ to reach perineal area and feet

Dressing: Seated in chair with arms, min Ⓐ to maintain dynamic balance when bending, mod Ⓐ to initiate donning bra, and max Ⓐ to reach feet. Verbal cues needed for sequencing and environmental orientation
Toileting: Verbal cues to flush, min Ⓐ to obtain tissue and manage clothing
Transfers: CGA with verbal cues for safety/proper arm placement sit to stand; min Ⓐ from low surfaces
Bed Mobility: Rolls & supine ↔ sit SBA for safety
Standing Balance: static: CGA
Activity Tolerance: fair (3) (1-5 scale) <10 min tolerance to any activity with physical/mental challenges
Motor Planning/Perception: WFL
Cognition: Score of 17/30 on Mini-Mental State Exam. Sequencing problems during dressing tasks noted. Client could not attach bra in back and required verbal cues to attach in front.
UE AROM: WFL for all Ⓑ UE movements except: abd, int/ext. rotation of Ⓛ shoulder lack ¼ range
UE Strength: Grip: Ⓡ 42#.; Ⓛ 21#. Pinch: Ⓡ palmar 14#; Ⓡ lateral 15#; Ⓛ palmar 6#; Ⓛ lateral 8#
Manual Muscle Test: All movements 4/5 except Ⓛ elbow ext. 3/5, thumb opposition and abduction 3+/5
Sensation: Ⓛ UE: Light touch, pain, temperature intact; stereognosis 3/5; Ⓡ UE all intact

A: Client's poor problem-solving skills (trying to doff pants prior to doffing shoes/socks and inability to initiate an alternative way to don bra) and the need for verbal cues to initiate some ADL tasks limit her ability to manage her basic and instrumental ADL activities Ⓘ. Decreased AROM and strength in the Ⓛ UE along with slow response to cognitive tasks, decreased ability to sequence tasks, and decreased short-term memory are safety concerns in an independent living situation. Client would benefit from environmental cues to orient her to environment, facilitation of problem solving and sequencing activities, and activities to increase strength in the Ⓛ UE. Rehab potential is good for modified Ⓘ in ADL activities.

P: OT for 45 minute sessions 5 X wk for 2 wks for sequencing during ADL tasks, problem-solving strategies, transfer training, activities to increase activity tolerance & strength in Ⓛ UE. Put calendar in client's room to increase orientation to month, day, and season. Evaluate ability to handle emergency situations.

Alice Altruism, OTR/L

Intervention Planning

The "A," or assessment, is a summary of deficits or problems that the OT determines from the initial evaluation. It can be in a narrative (paragraph) format but is often written as a numbered list of problems (called a *problem list*). Problems are defined as areas of occupation that are not within functional limits that will be addressed in treatment. Problem statements should include an underlying factor (performance skill, client factor, contextual limitation, etc.) and a related area of occupation. The best problem statements give a way of measuring the extent of the problem (such as "needs max assist" or "needs verbal cues"). Also remember that those who use our services are more than an assist level, so our statements should reflect what the client is **unable to do** or **needs assistance in doing** rather than saying that the client **is** a particular assist level. Instead of a narrative format as shown in the evaluation for Polly Payshent, the assessment can be written as a problem list.

Problem List

1.   Client needs min to max physical assist and verbal cues to dress and bathe self due to ↓ AROM, activity tolerance, and ability to sequence the task.

2.   Client's lack of orientation to environment and inability to problem solve create safety concerns with ADL and home management.

3.   Client needs CGA to min assist with functional mobility and transfers 2° decreased dynamic standing balance and decreased cognitive functions.

4.   Fair activity tolerance limits ability to manage BADLs and home management tasks.

5.   Moderately decreased left hand strength limits grip and prehension for grooming and hygiene tasks.

6.   Min AROM deficits in left shoulder limit client's ability to fasten bra and wash her back.

Worksheet 14-1
Initial Evaluation Report

Use this worksheet to help you compare the initial evaluation in this chapter to AOTA's recommended criteria. You can also use this worksheet to compare a "real" evaluation report to AOTA's criteria.

Background Data

Criteria	How Does the Evaluation Comply With the Criteria?
Are all of the following present: name, date of birth, gender? Are all applicable diagnoses listed?	
Is it clear who referred the client to OT, on what date, and what services were requested?	
Is the funding source listed for this client?	
Is anticipated length of stay indicated for this client?	
Why is the client seeking occupational therapy services?	
Are there any secondary problems, preexisting conditions, contraindications, or precautions that will impact therapy?	

Occupational History and Profile

Is there an occupational history/profile? Is it adequate?	
Which areas of occupation are currently successful and which are problematic?	
What factors hinder the client's performance in areas of occupation? What factors support performance in areas of occupation?	
What are the client's priorities? What does the client hope to gain from OT?	
What areas of occupation will be targeted for intervention? Do these match the client's priorities?	
What are the targeted outcomes?	

Results of the Assessment

What types of assessments were used?	
What were the results of the assessments?	
What client factors, contextual aspects, and activity demands are identified as needing attention?	
What factors (strengths, supports) facilitate the client's occupational performance?	
Are there other areas that need to be assessed that are not listed?	
Is OT appropriate for this client? Why or why not?	

Morreale, M. J., & Borcherding, S. (2013). *The OTA's guide to documentation: Writing SOAP notes (3rd ed.).* Thorofare, NJ: SLACK Incorporated.

Intervention Plan Guidelines

The assessment is the basis upon which the OT establishes the intervention plan. The therapist collaborates with the client (along with the family or significant other when appropriate) to prioritize the problems and establish an intervention plan to achieve desired outcomes. According to *Guidelines for Documentation of Occupational Therapy* (AOTA, 2008a), the intervention plan should include appropriate long- and short-term goals, the type of approach, methods or interventions to achieve those goals, the frequency and duration of treatment, and recommendations for other services or specialized treatments. It is oriented toward the client's quality of life and ultimate success in fulfilling life roles. The intervention plan must show the need for skilled occupational therapy and be realistic; that is, it must have a good chance of success in a reasonable period of time.

Estimating Rehabilitation Potential

Rehab potential is normally stated as good or excellent for the goals the OT establishes. If it is not good or excellent for the client, then a smaller more incremental goal must be selected. There is not much point in setting and working toward goals that do not have a good chance of being accomplished. Estimating rehab potential as guarded, fair, or poor is a red flag to reviewers, and they may be reluctant to set aside health care dollars for someone who is not likely to benefit from occupational therapy services. Rehab potential does not mean independence. It simply means potential to reach the goals the OT has set or potential for the client to make significant change. If a client's condition has a poor prognosis, such as cancer or Alzheimer's disease, goals might be established regarding what the caregiver needs to achieve to care for the client, such as ability to implement a home program of PROM, transfer or position the client properly, or safely feed a client who has dysphagia.

Expected Frequency and Duration

The frequency and duration of occupational therapy will vary according to physician orders, diagnosis, individual client needs and circumstances, payment source, and facility guidelines (Gateley & Borcherding, 2012). For example, in acute care, rehabilitation clients with a THR or CVA might be seen once or twice daily until discharge, but the length of sessions may vary depending on what the client can tolerate. Clients with general medical conditions such as pneumonia or another illness might only require one to two sessions for equipment recommendations or safety instructions prior to discharge home (Gateley & Borcherding, 2012). In an inpatient rehabilitation center, clients are typically seen once or twice daily for a total of 60 to 90 minutes for several weeks. Outpatients might be seen in occupational therapy two to three times weekly for 30 to 60 minutes for one or two sessions, a few weeks, or even several months for complex situations. Children in a school system receive occupational therapy based on what is delineated in the IEP. This might entail only a few occupational therapy sessions for consultation or ongoing therapy several times a week or month for the duration of the school year.

Selecting Intervention Strategies

Occupational therapy is a dynamic process of creative problem solving with each client in each area of occupation. What is meaningful to one client may not be to another. Even a very basic task such as dressing may not seem meaningful to some clients. A person with quadriplegia who has a personal attendant, for example, may never need to dress himself and may consider it an enormous waste of time to be required to learn to do so. However, he may be very motivated to learn to hold a mouth stick in order to engage in computer tasks for vocational retraining. Some clients will never need to balance a checkbook, while others may not be able to return to living independently without this skill. The occupational therapy practitioner asks questions like the following:

- What do you want to be able to do?
- What keeps you from being able to do that?
- What are the possible options for making that happen?

The options for intervention strategies may include teaching new skills or patterns, working to increase client factors (strength, range, and endurance), or modifying the environment (context). Occupational therapy practitioners consider doing things in many different or creative ways and try to make activities meaningful and purposeful to the client.

The treatment media used by occupational therapy is also different from that used by other disciplines. Occupational therapy practitioners often use common household objects to accomplish functional tasks. For example, the client's own clothing is a common treatment media. The clothes may be used for dressing to teach the client to don clothing, for folding in order to be doing a meaningful activity while increasing standing tolerance, for sorting colors for laundry, or for hanging in a closet to increase AROM at the shoulder. The approach would depend upon what the client will need to do in the expected discharge environment. An experienced OT or OTA can creatively find many different uses for common household objects. The same net ball that is used to wash dishes may be used for squeezing to develop grip strength, for tactile stimulation, or for throwing to develop UE range of motion. Let us look at the intervention plan for Polly Payshent, which includes the goals and methods to achieve those goals.

Intervention Plan

Problem #1: Client needs min to max physical assist and verbal cues to dress self due to ↓ AROM and strength, activity tolerance, and ability to sequence the task.

Long-term goal: Client will be able to dress with SBA and <3 verbal cues after set-up within 2 weeks.

Short-term goals:	Interventions:
Client will don bra modified Ⓘ using adapted technique within 3 days.	• Teach adaptive techniques. • Post picture of how to don bra correctly using adapted technique. • Reinforce correct responses. • Teach strengthening program for UE.
Client will don shoes and socks modified Ⓘ using adapted technique and a long shoe horn within 5 days.	• Provide long shoe horn and instruct client in correct use. • Instruct in adapted techniques for donning shoes and socks. • Post picture of adapted technique and long shoe horn being used to don shoes. • Instruct in using affected side as a functional assist in dressing. • Expand exercise program to include AROM.
Client will sequence dressing tasks correctly 3/3 tries within 1½ weeks.	• Verbalize steps before beginning to dress. • Verbalize steps while dressing. • Post list of steps for client to follow. • Take rest breaks as needed for activity tolerance.

Problem #2: Client's lack of orientation to environment and inability to problem solve create safety concerns with ADLs and home management.

Long-term goal: When asked, client will correctly use calendar, schedule, clock, and emergency information posted on wall within 2 weeks.

Short-term goals:	Interventions:
Client will identify time, date, and situation correctly when asked within 1 week.	• Post calendar, schedule, and emergency information near clock in client's room. • Instruct family, nursing staff, and other therapy staff to ask client date, time, and situation several times daily and to reinforce correct responses.
Client will be able to follow a daily schedule with <2 verbal cues within 1 to 2 weeks.	• Post daily schedule on wall near clock. • Cue client to look at schedule to determine what she should be doing at any given time.
Client will correctly problem solve responses to emergency situations with 90% accuracy within 2 weeks.	• Provide situations for client to problem solve, progressing from easy to more complex. • Provide telephone directory or other props as needed for problem solving.

Problem #3: Client's fair activity tolerance, decreased dynamic standing balance, and decreased cognitive functions necessitates CGA to min assist for functional mobility and transfers.

Long-term goal: Client will be able to perform functional transfers safely in bedroom and bathroom with modified Ⓘ.

Short-term goals:	Interventions:
Client will complete toilet transfers with modified Ⓘ within 2 weeks.	• Instruct client in use of grab bars and raised toilet seat. • Recommend purchase and installation of grab bar and raised toilet seat. • Post list of steps for client to follow and verbalize steps. • Implement grooming activities standing at sink to improve dynamic standing balance and endurance.
Client will perform commode transfers with SBA within 1 week.	• Place commode next to bed. • Recommend a commode be placed next to bed at home for use during the night. • Implement upper body AROM exercises while standing to improve dynamic standing balance and endurance.
Client will perform transfers EOB ↔ standing with SBA within 1 week.	• Instruct client in bed mobility and transfers. • Post list of steps for client to follow and verbalize steps. • Implement exercise band strengthening program while standing to improve dynamic standing balance and endurance.

Client to participate in OT for 45-minute sessions 5 X wk for 2 wks until anticipated discharge to her home. Will set up meeting with client's daughter to discuss equipment needs for home.

Alice Altruism, OTR/L

Worksheet 14-2
Intervention Plan

Use this worksheet to help you compare the intervention plan in this chapter to AOTA's recommended criteria. You can also use this worksheet to compare a "real" intervention plan to AOTA's criteria.

Criteria	How Does the Intervention Plan Comply With the Criteria?
Are specific occupational therapy interventions identified?	
Are the intervention goals and objectives measurable and realistic?	
Are the goals and objectives directly related to the client's occupational role performance?	
What is the anticipated frequency/duration of services?	
What is the discontinuation criteria or expected outcomes?	
What is the anticipated discharge location?	
What is the anticipated plan for follow-up care?	
Where will service be provided?	

Morreale, M. J., & Borcherding, S. (2013). *The OTA's guide to documentation: Writing SOAP notes (3rd ed.).* Thorofare, NJ: SLACK Incorporated.

Choosing Activities for Your Intervention Session

OTA students and novice practitioners often become anxious when their supervisors ask them to come up with specific treatment ideas for clients. You might wonder how you can even begin to think of appropriate activities to target the client's needs when the client has so many issues. You might be unsure as to what to work on first or how you can achieve all the goals in such a limited time. While you will certainly collaborate with your occupational therapy supervisor, you are also expected to think creatively and independently and to use your professional skills as an OTA to select appropriate treatment media or techniques. **The OT's intervention plan is your guide**. It spells out the areas to work on and the approaches to achieve those goals. For example, if a goal states, *"Client will be able to button half-inch buttons with modified Ⓘ using buttonhook,"* then your intervention session would include providing your client with a buttonhook and instructing the client how to use it. You would have the client practice buttoning and unbuttoning ½" buttons with the adaptive device. You could choose to do this on a button board or have the client practice on his shirt. A good occupational therapy activity combines working on several goals at once. If that same client also had the goal, *"Client will demonstrate increased activity tolerance for BADLs by standing 10 minutes at sink during grooming,"* you could have the client stand while practicing use of the buttonhook. Perhaps the client had a third goal, *"Client will increase strength of Ⓡ UE by one muscle grade in order to carry a laundry basket."* You might put a weighted cuff around the client's wrist while the client is standing and using the buttonhook. You have now worked on three goals with one treatment activity. Let us look at another example. Suppose the occupational therapy intervention plan had the following goals:

1. *Client will demonstrate improved decision-making skills for IADLs by planning a 2-course meal for OT cooking group with min verbal cues within 2 weeks.*

2. *Client will demonstrate organizational skills needed to complete IADLs within appropriate time periods within 3 weeks.*

3. *Client will demonstrate improved social interaction skills by asking a peer for assistance in OT group without prompting within 2 weeks.*

Mini Worksheet 14-3
Choosing Activities

How could you work on these goals at the same time? What would your treatment activities be? Compare your ideas with the suggestions that follow.

Morreale, M. J., & Borcherding, S. (2013). *The OTA's guide to documentation: Writing SOAP notes (3rd ed.).* Thorofare, NJ: SLACK Incorporated.

You might begin by having your client discuss ideas for the meal, have him look through a cookbook, or having him ask others in the group for ideas while he makes the final decision, all while giving verbal cues or encouragement as needed. The client then can prepare the meal in the occupational therapy cooking group. You can provide the opportunity for the client to ask others in the group to assist with some of the steps so it can be completed within the allotted time frame. This would integrate all of the goals at the same time and would be a good occupational therapy intervention.

Try creating another treatment scenario for the following goals in the OT's intervention plan:

1. *Student will be able to open all containers and wrappers Ⓘ for his lunch at school.*

2. *In order to perform bimanual classroom tasks, student will use Ⓛ hand spontaneously as a functional assist 5/5 opportunities.*

3. *Student will attend to classroom tasks for 10-minute periods with only one verbal cue for redirection.*

Mini Worksheet 14-4
Choosing Activities—More Practice

How could you work on these goals at the same time? What would your treatment activities be?

Now that you understand the initial evaluation process, you can begin to choose appropriate, realistic, and meaningful activities for your clients. Good occupational therapy activities often combine working on several goals at once to effectively achieve desired outcomes within the shortest time possible.

Morreale, M. J., & Borcherding, S. (2013). *The OTA's guide to documentation: Writing SOAP notes (3rd ed.).* Thorofare, NJ: SLACK Incorporated.

Chapter 15

Goals and Interventions

Occupational therapy goals must be written in functional, measurable, observable, and action-oriented terms. They must be realistic for the client, appropriate for the practice setting, and able to be achieved in a reasonable amount of time. Goals are initially formulated in the OT's intervention plan and must reflect the functional outcomes that the client hopes to gain from occupational therapy. Although improving underlying client factors or biomechanical components may be essential to achieving a desired functional outcome, those are much less important to a third-party payer than what the client can actually do. The OTA will implement day-to-day treatment activities and various methods to achieve the outcomes outlined in the intervention plan. What transpires during the intervention session is recorded in a SOAP note. As noted in Chapter 10, the "P" part of the SOAP note could end with a goal statement, depending on facility or payer requirements, but this is not always needed. Progress notes may also incorporate goals. It is not necessary to repeatedly restate goals that are already written in the initial evaluation. You will be aligning your treatment to the established intervention plan and, with the OT's supervision, might write goals to reflect the steps along the way that your client needs to achieve desired outcomes.

Goals in an intervention plan are called **long-term goals** (LTG) or outcomes. These are usually what the client hopes to accomplish by the time of discharge. The OT will typically create at least one LTG for each problem identified in the occupational therapy evaluation. Time frames for LTGs will vary significantly according to the type of practice setting and the client's circumstances. **Short-term goals** (STG), also called *objectives*, are the incremental goals or sub-steps that are met while progressing toward the long-term or discharge goals. For example, if the LTG is:

> *In order to perform job without injury, client will be able to move 35# objects needed for work from table to counter without ↑ in pain by 2/18/13.*

An STG might be:

> *Client will be able to lift 10 # objects needed for work without ↑ in pain by 2/5/13.*

There may be STGs (objectives) for each LTG. For example, suppose you are treating a client who is a 49-year-old postal worker who sustained a Ⓡ CVA a few days ago and has Ⓛ side hemiplegia. The OT's evaluation states that he has verbal abilities and intact mental functions. The intervention plan has identified a goal of independent upper body dressing by 3/25/13. This will require skilled instruction and the correct adaptive equipment.

A series of short-term goals must be established:

1. *Client will be able to maintain dynamic sitting balance at EOB for >5 minutes while reaching for clothing at arm's length, within three treatment sessions.*

2. *By the 6th treatment session, client will demonstrate increased activity tolerance for >10 minutes of dressing while sitting at edge of bed.*

Morreale MJ, Borcherding S.
The OTA's Guide to Documentation:
Writing SOAP Notes, Third Edition (pp 141-153).
© 2013 SLACK Incorporated.

3. *Client will be able to don shirt sitting EOB using the over-the-head method by 3/15/13.*

4. *Client will be able to button shirt with modified Ⓘ using a buttonhook by 3/18/13.*

5. *While sitting EOB, client will demonstrate independence in upper body dressing by 3/25/13.*

As you can see, each of these STGs is measurable, observable, and client-action oriented. The first four STGs are steps to reach the ultimate LTG (Figure 15-1).

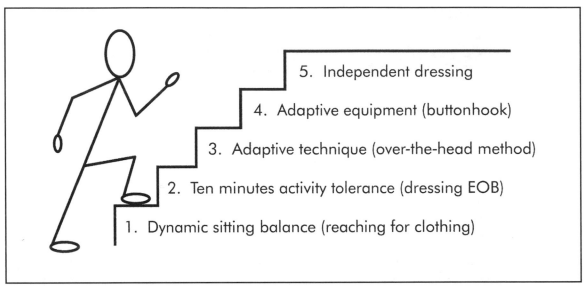

Figure 15-1. Steps to the ultimate LTG.

An intervention plan is always a work in progress, and you and the OT will collaborate to provide the most appropriate care. Unexpected events and conditions can impact the progress your client will be able to make toward his or her goals. The OT will modify the intervention plan as needed (based upon your feedback), as it is not useful to continue with a plan that is not working. In order to write appropriate goals and objectives in a way that can be measured, the elements to be included are very specific. The COAST format, developed by Gateley & Borcherding (2012) is a useful method as you are learning. The COAST format will help you to include all of the necessary components and can easily be adapted for the specific terminology and criteria used in different practice settings. Sometimes the order of the COAST elements may need to be changed slightly in order for your sentence to make sense. As long as all of the required elements are present, you can begin with any of the COAST elements—the client expectation, functional occupation, assist level, conditions, or timeline (Gateley & Borcherding, 2012).

Goal Writing: The COAST Method

C – Client	Client will perform
O – Occupation	What occupation?
A – Assist Level	With what level of assistance/independence?
S – Specific Condition	Under what conditions?
T – Timeline	By when?

Reprinted with permission from Gateley, C. A., & Borcherding, S. (2012). *Documentation manual for occupational therapy: Writing SOAP notes* (3rd ed.). Thorofare, NJ: SLACK Incorporated.

Now let us look at each of the COAST categories (Gateley & Borcherding, 2012).

C (Client)

When writing goals in occupational therapy, the **client** must be the main focus. The goal statement is **not** the place to tell what the OT or OTA will do. That goes later, under intervention strategies. The occupational therapy practitioner sets the expectation for what the client—not the OT or OTA—will achieve:

> ***The client will…***
>
> ***The client will*** *perform transfers w/c ↔ toilet with SBA by 1/4/13.*
>
> ***Child will*** *demonstrate ability to tie her shoes (Ⓘ) within 3 weeks.*

Use an appropriate action verb such as "*demonstrate,*" "*complete,*" or "*perform*" to indicate the client expectation (Gateley & Borcherding, 2012). In some instances, the goal might indicate what the parent or caregiver will achieve after your skilled instruction:

> *After skilled instruction,* ***parent will*** *demonstrate proper technique to position child for feeding by end of 2nd treatment session.*
>
> ***Client's spouse will*** *demonstrate ability to transfer client safely from bed ↔ commode following skilled instruction within 1 week.*

O (Occupation)

Goals should pertain to and specify **occupation** and directly relate to a problem that was identified in the occupational therapy intervention plan (Gateley & Borcherding, 2012). The ability to engage in occupation is the heart and core of occupational therapy practice. It should be the **first** thing you think of when writing goals, and it should be the goal statement's prime focus. For example:

> *Client will* ***don pullover sweater…***
>
> *Client will be able to* ***complete his morning medication regimen…***
>
> *The client will* ***perform a three-step cooking process…***

If your goal emphasizes a particular client factor or performance skill as an essential part of a desired occupation, be sure to include the area of occupation that this factor or skill will ultimately enable the client to do, such as, "*in order to return to work as a carpenter,*" "*in order to be able to be bathed by his caretakers,*" or "*in order to be able to write his name at school.*" The following is an example:

> ***In order to begin writing her name at school,*** *student will demonstrate ability to hold pencil with a static tripod grasp by 6/19/13.*

The occupation may go after the action if you prefer. For example:

> *Student will demonstrate ability to hold pencil with a static tripod grasp when* ***writing her name at school*** *by 6/19/13.*

A (Assist Level)

This part of the goal delineates the expected level of assistance that the client will achieve when performing the specific occupation. This includes quantifiable physical assistance levels or verbal, tactile, or visual cues. If your facility uses a specific outcome measure such as the Functional Independence Measure, it might be appropriate to incorporate those criteria into your goals (Gateley & Borcherding, 2012). Review Chapter 8 for various ways to describe assist levels. The following are some examples:

> *Client will complete shaving* ***with less than four verbal cues to attend to left side of face…***
>
> *Client will don pullover shirt* ***with min assist to place Ⓛ arm in sleeve…***
>
> *To demonstrate increased self-esteem for socialization, client will verbalize three positive attributes* ***with min verbal prompting*** *within 1 week.*

S (Specific Condition)

This represents additional criteria or conditions under which the client is expected to be able to perform the desired action such a compensatory technique, use of durable medical equipment/adaptive equipment, client position, location, etc. (Gateley & Borcherding, 2012). For example:

*Client will perform upper and lower body dressing Ⓘ, **taking less than three 60-second rest breaks** by 01/05/13.*

*In order to perform dressing, client will maintain static sitting balance Ⓘ on **edge of bed for three minutes** by 1/3/13.*

The conditions make your goal more specific. One of the most common mistakes in goal writing is omission of the conditions under which the activity is expected to be performed. Usually it is helpful to put the condition **after** the skill rather than before it, but sometimes you may want to start with the condition. For example,

***While standing at sink for 5 minutes**, client will demonstrate ability to wash and dry dishes with SBA by 2/20/2013.*

***Using a buttonhook**, client will button at least three buttons on her shirt modified Ⓘ by 4/1/13.*

Using both the "A" and the "S" will help ensure that your goal is measurable and will demonstrate gains that your client has achieved (Gateley & Borcherding, 2012). The following are some more examples:

- *with SBA using a grab bar*
- *with hand-over-hand assist while standing at blackboard*
- *Ⓘ while seated in wheelchair*
- *with two verbal cues using a daily planner*
- *with modified Ⓘ referring to a list of instructions*
- *independently with arm supported on laptray*
- *with visual demonstration in crafts group*
- *with modified independence using a timer*
- *mod Ⓐ without shortness of breath*
- *after set-up with one verbal cue for initiation*
- *min Ⓐ while seated upright in bed*

In some instances, it is acceptable to use only the "A" or the "S," but you must use at least one of them (Gateley & Borcherding, 2012). For example, a client may have independence in a particular task but difficulty performing it due to a specific client factor such as low endurance or pain. In that case, you could eliminate stating an implied independent assist level but still state the conditions (Gateley & Borcherding, 2012). In the following examples, the measurable criteria are factors such as pain level, activity tolerance, quality of the task, and amount of time needed.

*Client will carry laundry basket 20 feet with a **reported pain level of less than 5/10**.*

*Client will stand at stove 10 minutes to cook a meal **without shortness of breath**.*

*Student will demonstrate ability to carry lunch tray from cafeteria line to table **without spilling any items**.*

*Client will demonstrate improved decision-making skills by choosing one out of four possible projects **within 60 seconds** in OT craft group.*

Children sometimes exhibit a new behavior inconsistently before it is really established. Therefore, measurement used for children is more likely to reflect whether the behavior is established. For example,

*Kevin will use a Ⓡ pincer grasp to pick up and feed self 10 raisins **3/3 opportunities**.*

*Chrystal will demonstrate improved tolerance to tactile media as evidenced by self-initiation during art activities in **5/5 teacher reports**.*

*Student will demonstrate ability to open combination lock on locker within 60 seconds **4/5 opportunities**.*

*Student will maintain upright sitting posture during classroom writing time without verbal reminders in **3/3 observations**.*

You may find that some school settings use percentages in goals such as, *"Child will demonstrate ability to bring food to mouth with spoon without spilling 75% of the time by the end of school year."* However, it is more clear to say, *"Child will demonstrate ability to bring food to mouth with spoon without spilling 15/20 opportunities by the end of school year."* This way, anyone can observe the exact behavior and number of repetitions and determine if the criteria are met. Goals for children in public schools must be set in terms of a behavior that is needed in the classroom or school context. While you may be working on sensory integration as a treatment intervention, such as maintaining prone extension posture on a scooter board, it must be written in language that is educationally based, relating to performance in the classroom setting.

T (Timeline)

This is the time frame within which the goal is expected to be accomplished. In a practice setting where notes are written monthly, the goal would be what you hope to accomplish in the next month. In an acute care setting, it might be your goal for tomorrow. In a school setting, goals in the Individualized Education Program are considered annual goals with a time frame for the end of the school year. Benchmarks are then established to measure progress toward the annual goals. In a rehabilitation hospital or subacute unit, LTGs typically have time frames that coincide with the expected discharge date from the facility, which might only be a week or two. For example:

While seated on tub bench, client will demonstrate ability to bathe upper body with SBA…

- *…by the end of the next treatment session.*
- *…within 2 weeks.*
- *…within 1 month.*
- *…within three treatment sessions.*
- *…by expected discharge on 10/16/12.*

COAST Examples

C—Client will complete
O—setting the table
A—with SBA
S—using rolling walker and walker tray
T—within 1 week

C—Student will demonstrate ability to
O—open combination lock on locker
A—independently
S—and get to next class on time 5/5 opportunities
T—by the end of the school year

C—Child will
O—use left hand to stabilize paper when drawing
A—with min verbal cues
S—4/5 opportunities
T—within 1 month

C—Client will perform
O—toilet transfers
A—with min assist
S—using walker and adhering to total hip precautions
T—within 3 days

Client will perform all laundry tasks Ⓘ at laundromat by anticipated discharge on 3/13/13.

Student will be able to change into his gym clothes within 5 minutes 3/3 opportunities by the end of the school year.

Infant will be able to reach for a toy while supine by bringing Ⓡ UE to midline with min assist by 1/31/2013.

Other Considerations for Goals

Demonstrating Progress for Specific Performance Components and Client Factors

Sometimes, a performance skill or client factor needs to be emphasized in a goal to show that the client is making progress with specific deficits, particularly for clients with cognitive or behavioral problems. As noted with the COAST method, an occupation-based task should be clearly identified in a goal along with the assist level, specific condition, and timeline. The following template is useful when particular performance skills or client factors must be addressed to prepare the client for function and demonstrate progress. However, the order of these components may sometimes need to be changed for the goal to make sense:

Client will demonstrate _____ _____ _____
(use words such as improved   (performance skill   (in order to do what occupation)
or an increase of)   or client factor)

_____ _____.
(assist level and/or specific condition)   (time frame—by when)

Client will demonstrate improved time management skills for BADLs by completing a shower Ⓘ in 15 minutes or less within 1 week.

Client will demonstrate improved attention to Ⓛ side when eating by locating all utensils and food items on Ⓛ side of meal tray with three verbal cues or less within 3 days.

To reach clothes hanging in closet, client will demonstrate an increase of 20° shoulder flexion within 2 weeks.

Infant will demonstrate improved proximal stability for play by maintaining prone while supported on elbows for 5 minutes within 1 month.

Student will demonstrate improved bilateral integration during classroom tasks by using both hands spontaneously to place paper in folder 5/5 opportunities by the end of the school year.

Within 3 days, client will demonstrate increased assertiveness by asking a peer to share condiments during 3/3 meals without verbal prompting.

In order to manage laundry, client will demonstrate improved dexterity to manipulate coins and insert in coin-operated washing machine Ⓘ by anticipated discharge on 9/13/12.

Skilled Occupational Therapy

It is important to remember that your documentation must demonstrate a clear need for skilled occupational therapy. Once a client reaches the level of minimal assistance, the changes become more subtle, and may lead to denial of payment unless you specify the necessity of skilled occupational therapy. For example, dressing with minimal assistance does not necessarily indicate a need for skilled occupational therapy. However, documenting interventions such as *"minimal assistance with verbal instruction for over-the-head method of donning of shirt"* could justify skilled occupational therapy. Client goals must also reflect the reasonable, necessary, and skilled services that occupational therapy practitioners provide. In addition, the client's priorities must be addressed within the short time frames allowed for therapy. For example, a client residing in a nursing home may benefit more from goals that address independent wheelchair mobility, feeding, or ability to manage eyeglasses, rather than a goal that might only improve lower body dressing from moderate to minimum assistance. Choosing what kind of goal to use and the specific criteria depend upon the individual's unique needs in addition to the type of setting and the funding source. As previously noted, goals in a school setting must be educationally related. Physical rehabilitation goals for adult and elderly clients should generally focus on BADLs, work, or IADLs, as leisure activities are not typically considered a priority by Medicare and other payers. Goals in early intervention normally address developmental milestones. Regardless of the setting, goals should be client-centered and occupation-based, written in measurable objective terms, and include a timeline (Gateley & Borcherding, 2012).

The Client Is not an Assist Level

Consider the following goal, which needs some improvement:

Client will be min Ⓐ in dressing LEs in 10 days.

This goal needs to be written in terms of what the client **needs** rather than stating that he **will be** a particular assist level. It is a small item that shows more respect to word the goal statement so that it acknowledges that the client is more than his ability to dress himself.

Specify the conditions under which the client will dress himself (including what parts of the task need assistance) rather than that he will dress only his upper and lower extremities. For example:

Client will be able to don lower body garments sitting EOB with min Ⓐ to pull pants and underwear over hips within 10 days.

Numbering the Short-Term Goals

Some occupational therapy practitioners number each STG. For example:

STG #1: *Consumer will demonstrate independence in laundry skills by selecting and inserting correct amount of money in coin-operated washing machine by 4/25/13.*
STG #2: *Consumer will demonstrate ↑ laundry skills by selecting proper cycles on washing machine by 4/25/13.*

In subsequent SOAP notes, the OT or OTA can refer to those numbered goals, providing a clear indication of the progress achieved. For example:

A: *STG #1: met. STG #2: Consumer requires min verbal cues 50% of the time to select proper wash cycles for white and dark clothes.*
P: *Consumer will continue skilled instruction in IADLs until anticipated discharge in 4 weeks. At the time of discharge, consumer will be able to manage all laundry tasks Ⓘ at laundromat.*

DO NOT use participation in treatment as a goal. For example:

Client will do 20 reps of shoulder ladder with 1# wt. in order to ↑ endurance to become more Ⓘ in ADLs.

In a goal such as this, specify the amount of ↑ endurance you hope or expect to see. For example:

Client will be able to participate in assembly line task >10 minutes without rest breaks.

Rather than saying:

Client will use therapy putty to ↑ hand strength by 5 lbs.

It is better to say:

Client will ↑ hand strength by 5 lbs in order to be able to open jars.

Rather than saying:

Client will play a board game with other clients.

It is better to say:

Client will demonstrate improved self-confidence by Ⓘ initiating a leisure activity with peers.

Examples of Appropriate Goal Statements for Different Situations

Basic Activities of Daily Living

Dressing

- *To prepare for recess, child will be able to manage zipper on coat with use of zipper pull within 1 month.*
- *In order to tie shoelaces Ⓘ, patient will demonstrate Ⓡ thumb MP flexion of no less than 50° within 2 weeks.*

Hygiene

- *Patient will complete grooming and hygiene activities with a reported pain level of <3/10 within three treatment sessions.*

Worksheet 15-2
Writing Goals That Are Client-Centered, Occupation-Based, and Measurable

Review the scenarios below and write goals that are client-centered, occupation-based, measurable, time-limited, and realistic. Goals are established with the client (under the supervision of the OT), so assume for this practice sheet that you have already collaborated with the client and your supervisor.

1. Your client, Maria, has difficulty with IADL tasks because she is unable to attend to task for more than a few minutes. Because she enjoys cooking and plans to resume cooking after discharge, you have been working with her in the kitchen. You would like to see her able to attend to task for 10 minutes by the time she is discharged next week. Write a goal to increase Maria's attention span.

C _____
   (Client will perform)

O _____
   (Occupation)

A _____
   (Assist level)

S _____
   (Specific conditions)

T _____
   (Timeline—by when?)

2. Now write a goal for Maria to be able to follow directions so that she can read the back of a boxed meal, and eventually a recipe, when she is cooking.

C _____
   (Client will perform)

O _____
   (Occupation)

A _____
   (Assist level)

S _____
   (Specific conditions)

T _____
   (Timeline—by when?)

3. Bill is having trouble performing dressing tasks after his stroke. You have been teaching him an over-the-head method for putting on his shirt and have given him a buttonhook to use. Write a dressing goal for Bill.

C _____
   (Client will perform)

O _____
   (Occupation)

A _____
   (Assist level)

S _____
   (Specific conditions)

T _____
   (Timeline—by when?)

Morreale, M. J., & Borcherding, S. (2013). *The OTA's guide to documentation: Writing SOAP notes (3rd ed.)*. Thorofare, NJ: SLACK Incorporated.

Worksheet 15-2 (continued)
Writing Goals That Are Client-Centered, Occupation-Based, and Measurable

Review the scenarios below and write goals that are client-centered, occupation-based, measurable, time-limited, and realistic. Goals are established with the client (under the supervision of the OT), so assume for this practice sheet that you have already collaborated with the client and your supervisor.

4. Susan has significant weakness and desires to be able to care for her 4-month-old child and also go back to work as a receptionist. Write a goal to increase her activity tolerance. Anticipated discharge is in 2 weeks.

    C _____
    (Client will perform)

    O _____
    (Occupation)

    A _____
    (Assist level)

    S _____
    (Specific conditions)

    T _____
    (Timeline—by when?)

5. Alberto wants to live independently in the community, but he lacks basic money management skills. Write a goal for Alberto to improve his money management skills.

    C _____
    (Client will perform)

    O _____
    (Occupation)

    A _____
    (Assist level)

    S _____
    (Specific conditions)

    T _____
    (Timeline—by when?)

6. Katelyn has become increasingly more depressed over the past several weeks and was admitted after a suicide attempt. You estimate that you will have her in groups for 1 week. You would like to see her mood change in that week. Write a goal that is occupation-based and will indicate an improved mood.

    C _____
    (Client will perform)

    O _____
    (Occupation)

    A _____
    (Assist level)

    S _____
    (Specific conditions)

    T _____
    (Timeline—by when?)

Morreale, M. J., & Borcherding, S. (2013). *The OTA's guide to documentation: Writing SOAP notes (3rd ed.).* Thorofare, NJ: SLACK Incorporated.

Worksheet 15-3

Writing Goals—Developmental Disability

Jake is an 18-year-old male with a developmental disability. He has just moved into a group home with five other clients. Jake exhibits mild to moderate cognitive impairment but can perform personal ADLs with supervision and occasional assistance. Muscle tone is minimally hypotonic, but there are no other physical limitations. He has a fair frustration tolerance and occasionally exhibits some aggressive behavior. The plan is to improve Jake's social skills and allow him to be more independent in the group home and community.

Using the information in the above scenario, write a short-term occupation-based goal for each of the categories listed below. Make sure your goals are appropriate and realistic for this particular practice setting, keeping in mind the client's abilities and expected functional gains.

1. Instrumental ADL—meal preparation: _____

   _____

2. Instrumental ADL—household chore: _____

   _____

3. Instrumental ADL—shopping: _____

   _____

4. Instrumental ADL—money management/functional math skill: _____

   _____

5. Communication/interaction skills: _____

   _____

6. Prevocational skills: _____

   _____

7. Temporal organization/time management: _____

   _____

Worksheet 15-4
Goal Writing—Functional BADL Components

There are instances when specific performance skills or client factors must be emphasized in goals to prepare the client for function and demonstrate progress. Create a client in your mind and consider the BADL task of tooth brushing. Using the client factors and performance skills below, write goals for the occupation of tooth brushing that address each listed component. Remember to include the assist level, specific condition, and timeline.

BADL: Brushing Teeth

1. Fine-motor skills: _____

   _____

2. Hand strength: _____

   _____

3. Standing balance: _____

   _____

4. Unilateral inattention: _____

   _____

5. Elbow range of motion: _____

   _____

6. Problem solving: _____

   _____

7. Spatial relations: _____

   _____

Morreale, M. J., & Borcherding, S. (2013). *The OTA's guide to documentation: Writing SOAP notes (3rd ed.)*. Thorofare, NJ: SLACK Incorporated.

Electronic records usually eliminate the need to reenter the client's identifying or demographic information each time an occupational therapy note is created (Herbold, 2010). That information is typically present when the existing file is opened. In hospital and nursing homes using printed records, the client's identifying or demographic information is usually stamped onto each page of the health record using an addressograph card. In those situations, it is also unnecessary for the OT or OTA to rewrite that same information on the same page.

Contact Notes

Contact, visit, or treatment notes are used to document each encounter or occupational therapy session. Besides face-to-face contact with the client, these notes can also include pertinent telephone conversations; e-mail communication; or meetings with the client, family/caregiver, other professionals, or service providers (AOTA, 2008a). As previously discussed in Chapter 11, notes are also written stating why a scheduled session did not take place, ended prematurely, or involved unusual circumstances. In situations such as home health or acute care, formal contact notes are typically written in the health record each time a client is seen. In situations such as school settings or some skilled nursing facilities, occupational therapy practitioners might keep attendance records, logs, billing sheets, or informal contact notes, which are used for the purpose of writing a summary of progress later on. Practice settings vary regarding exact format and content for treatment notes. Your facility or agency will normally supply you with designated printed or computerized forms to use. The *Guidelines for Documentation of Occupational Therapy* (AOTA 2008a), suggests the following criteria for contact notes:

1. Documents contacts between the client and the occupational therapy practitioner. Records the types of interventions used and client's response. Includes telephone contacts, interventions, and meetings with others.
2. Suggested content with examples include
   a. *Client information*—name/agency, date of birth, gender, diagnosis, precautions, and contraindications
   b. *Therapy log*—date, type of contact, names/positions of persons involved, summary or significant information communicated during contacts, client attendance and participation in intervention, reason service is missed, types of interventions used, client's response, environmental or task modification, assistive or adaptive devices used or fabricated, statement of any training education or consultation provided, and the persons present

Reprinted with permission from American Occupational Therapy Association. (2008a). Guidelines for documentation of occupational therapy. *American Journal of Occupational Therapy, 62*(6), 684-690.

The following is an example of an acute care contact note that incorporates the AOTA guidelines:

Healthy Hospital
Acute Care Unit
Occupational Therapy Contact Note

Client: Klyent, Karl   **DOB**: 11/10/1931   **Health record #**: 123456
Dx: COPD   **Sex**: Male   **Physician**: Dr. Will Heelue
Precautions/Contraindications: Maintain O_2 levels at 95% to 100%
Date: 4/14/13   **Time**: 8:30 AM
  S: Client reported, "I feel fair today. I had a long night."
  O: In ICU, client participated in bedside session for instruction in ADL tasks and to increase activity tolerance. Client required mod Ⓐ supine → sit. Upon sitting EOB, O_2 saturation dropped to ~85%. Client required min Ⓐ to return to supine. After ~2 minutes, O_2 levels returned to ~95%. With head of bed raised and ADL set-up, client washed face, combed hair, and brushed teeth with O_2 levels ~95% without rest breaks.
  A: Client appears more motivated to attempt therapy session as compared to his refusal of therapy yesterday. Activity tolerance still limited due to O_2 saturation levels upon exertion, which limits ability to participate in self-care tasks. Client would benefit from instruction in energy conservation as well as correct positioning to ↓ exertion and ↑ activity tolerance for ADL tasks.
  P: Continue skilled OT daily for 5 days or until discharge from acute care to ↑ activity tolerance and Ⓘ in ADL tasks. Client will complete grooming modified Ⓘ sitting EOB with rest breaks as needed within 3 treatment sessions.

Vera Veracity, COTA—Kimberly Kindness, OTR/L

Worksheet 16-1
Treatment, Visit, or Contact Notes

Use this worksheet as you are learning to write treatment notes. You may also use this worksheet to compare a "real" treatment note to AOTA's recommended criteria.

Criteria	How Does Your Note Comply With the Criteria?
Does the note state the client's full name and identifying number?	
Is information relating to the client's diagnosis and precautions/contraindications specified?	
Is the facility or agency identified?	
Are the date (and time, if needed) of the contact indicated?	
Is the note identified as occupational therapy?	
Is the type of note indicated?	
Are the names (and positions, if appropriate) of the persons involved in the contact specified?	
Does the note state the type of contact and purpose of the encounter?	
Is there a summary of the interventions implemented or information communicated during the contact (e.g., modification of the task or environment, assistive/adaptive devices used, education, training, or consultation provided), and indication of specific persons present?	
Is the client's participation in the contact (or the reason service was missed) indicated?	
Are all abbreviations and terminology standard and acceptable for the setting?	
Are errors corrected properly?	
Is a line drawn through any blank spaces?	
Is the note signed (and cosigned if needed)?	
Are professional credentials indicated next to the signature?	

Morreale, M. J., & Borcherding, S. (2013). *The OTA's guide to documentation: Writing SOAP notes (3rd ed.)*. Thorofare, NJ: SLACK Incorporated.

Progress Notes

Progress notes are written on a regularly scheduled basis, which might be weekly, every 2 weeks, or monthly. The facility determines the specific time frame by considering the guidelines set forth by accrediting agencies and primary payers. Progress notes provide a summary of the intervention process and record the client's progress toward goals. The *Guidelines for Documentation of Occupational Therapy* (AOTA, 2008a) list the following criteria for the content of a progress report:

1. Summarizes intervention process and documents client's progress toward goals achievement. Includes new data collected; modifications of treatment plan; and statement of need for continuation, discontinuation, or referral.

2. Suggested content with examples include

   a. *Client information*—name/agency, date of birth, gender, diagnosis, precautions, and contraindications

   b. *Summary of services provided*—brief statement of frequency of services and length of time services have been provided; techniques and strategies used; environmental or task modifications provided; adaptive equipment or orthotics provided; medical, educational, or other pertinent client updates; client's response to occupational therapy services; and programs or training provided to the client or caregivers

   c. *Current client performance*—client's progress toward the goals and client's performance in areas of occupations

   d. *Plan or recommendations*—recommendations and rationale as well as client's input to changes or continuation of plan

Reprinted with permission from American Occupational Therapy Association. (2008a). Guidelines for documentation of occupational therapy. *American Journal of Occupational Therapy, 62*(6), 684-690.

The following is an example of a progress note that incorporates the AOTA guidelines:

XYZ Behavioral Health Center
Occupational Therapy Progress Note

Client: Payshent, Patricia   **DOB**: 1/10/1951   **Health record #**: 54321
Dx: Depression   **Sex**: Female   **Physician**: Bea Well, MD
SOC: 10/01/12
Date: 10/12/2012

S: In assertion group on Wednesday, 10/10/12, client talked about how her life had taken a "downward spiral" since early September, and she had become more passive and less proactive in getting her needs met, although she had not been aware of it at the time.

O: Client attended assertion group 2/2, communication group 1/1, and IADL group 3/5 this week. She was on time to 4/6 groups without reminders, wearing neatly pressed clothing, makeup, and an ornament in her hair. In assertion group on Thursday, 10/11, she shared (without prompting) two stories about her usual way of dealing with retail situations. In communication group, she spontaneously answered one question addressed to the group as a whole, and in IADL group, she offered to assist another client with his checkbook.

A: Client's spontaneous actions in groups and willingness to share verbally indicate an improved mood this week. Her unprompted attendance is up this week from 2/8 to 6/8 groups. Her improved dress, hygiene, and makeup also indicate an improvement in mood from last week. Client would benefit from planning a structure for her days to prevent another "downward spiral" after discharge, and she has expressed willingness to work on this.
Goals #1: (assertion) and #2: (communication) are met as of this date.
Goal #3: (leisure skills) is continued through discharge on 10/14/12 pending formulation of a plan.
Goal #4: (parenting skills) was discontinued on 10/10/12.

P: Client to participate in groups for 2 more days, with discharge anticipated on 10/14/12. IADL group and individual session, if needed, will be used for preparing the structured plan for using her time. Client will prepare a plan including at least one planned leisure activity per day for at least 5 days out of 7 after discharge and will discuss it with her husband and social worker by discharge on 10/14/12.

Evan Empathy, COTA—Sharon Sympathetic, OTR/L

Worksheet 16-2
Progress Notes

Use this worksheet as you are learning to write progress notes. You may also use this worksheet to compare a "real" progress note to AOTA's recommended criteria.

Criteria	How Does Your Note Comply With the Criteria?
Does the note state the client's full name and identifying number?	
Has new data been obtained and presented?	
Does the note state pertinent client updates, problems, or changes to the intervention plan?	
Does the note indicate the frequency of services and how long services have been provided?	
Is information relating to the client's diagnosis and precautions/contraindications specified?	
Does the note indicate the client's response to occupational therapy services?	
Does the note indicate what progress the client is making toward his goals?	
Is the facility or agency identified?	
Is the date of the progress note specified?	
Is the note identified as occupational therapy?	
Is the type of note indicated?	
Does the note indicate what areas of occupation are being addressed?	
Does the note reflect the client's occupational performance?	
Is there a summary of techniques and strategies used? Does the note specify environmental modifications, assistive/adaptive devices, orthotics, or other skilled services provided?	
Does the note indicate the type of education, training, or consultation that has been provided and to whom?	
Does the note specify progress the client is making toward goals?	
Are recommendations indicated along with rationale?	
Does the note reflect the client's input to changes or continuation of the intervention plan?	
Are all abbreviations and terminology standard and acceptable for the setting?	
Are errors corrected properly?	
Is a line drawn through any blank spaces?	
Is the note signed (and cosigned if needed)?	
Are professional credentials indicated next to the signature?	

Morreale, M. J., & Borcherding, S. (2013). *The OTA's guide to documentation: Writing SOAP notes (3rd ed.).* Thorofare, NJ: SLACK Incorporated.

As you can see, contact notes and progress notes fit neatly into the SOAP format. Reevaluation reports, transition plans, and discharge summaries may also use a SOAP format but generally require more organization, analysis, intervention planning, and a broader base of knowledge. The OT is responsible for developing and documenting these documents. However, OTAs can participate in all aspects of the intervention process and can contribute to documentation at all stages under the OT's supervision (AOTA, 2009, 2010c). Therefore, we will take a brief look at reevaluations, transition plans, and discharge reports.

Reevaluation Reports

Practice settings vary regarding time frames for reevaluation. Clients might be reevaluated monthly, quarterly, or on an as-needed basis. The reevaluation is the responsibility of the OT, but certain functions might be delegated to the OTA (AOTA, 2010c). According to the *Guidelines for Documentation of Occupational Therapy* (AOTA, 2008a), the reevaluation report should include information about the client's condition along with a summary or update of issues, changes, or concerns that relate to the occupational profile. In addition, the tests that were given initially are readministered and the results are compared with the results of prior tests to determine the effectiveness of the treatment being provided. Revisions are then made to the goals and plans and new timelines are projected.

XYZ Hand Clinic
Occupational Therapy Department
Reevaluation Report

Name: Doe, Jane   **DOB**: 4/01/71   **Gender**: Female   **Record #**: 12345
Primary diagnosis: Osteoarthritis in Ⓑ CMC joints
Secondary diagnosis: None
Precautions/contraindications: None
Referring physician: B. Paynefree, MD   **Date of referral**: June 27, 2012
Reason for referral: Client is 1 month post surgery (LRTI) to the Ⓛ CMC joint and CTR
Date of initial evaluation: 7/5/2012
Date of reevaluation: 8/31/2012
Funding source: University insurance
Occupational profile: Jane is a 41-year-old Caucasian female who works as an administrative assistant in the English Department at the University. She lives alone in a small 2-story farmhouse 7 miles outside of town. The house is heated with wood that Jane cuts and stacks in the summer. Jane raises a large vegetable garden every year in addition to holding both a full-time job at the University and a part-time job in a department store. She began experiencing pain in the CMC joints of both hands approximately 3 years ago. She intends to continue her present living arrangement and both of her jobs. She was originally admitted to the outpatient hand clinic on July 5, 2012 at 1 month post surgery for hand rehabilitation following a successful Ⓛ LRTI and a carpal tunnel release. She is being reevaluated this date (8/31/12) to determine whether further OT services are needed.

S: Client initially reported continuous pain at a level of 3/10 and pain on overexertion of the Ⓛ hand at a level of 5/10, resulting in difficulty performing bilateral work and daily living tasks, as well as some tasks requiring left hand use. On this date, she reports no continuous pain and pain at a level of 1/10 when typing for more than 45 minutes without rest breaks.
Initial ability to engage in work/ADL/IADL tasks (by client report):
- Unable to use keyboard with all fingers of Ⓛ hand. Types with one finger on standard keyboard.
- Unable to grasp cylindrical objects smaller that 1½ inches (broom handle, toothpaste tube) due to ↓ AROM
- Unable to wear watch or rings on Ⓛ hand due to swelling
- Unable to turn door knob with Ⓛ hand to enter house when right hand is full.
- Unable to lift laundry basket and other items requiring Ⓑ UE use. Unable to lift purse or other items needed for IADL tasks with left hand

Current ability to engage in work/ADL/IADL tasks this date (by client report):
- Able to use new ergonomic keyboard for primary work task using all fingers
- Able to sweep the floors with a regular broom
- Able to fold laundry using Ⓑ hands
- Able to grasp small items needed for ADL and IADL tasks (toothpaste tube, key, lids), but not at prior level of function
- Able to turn doorknob if door is unlocked
- Able to hang out clothes on clothesline, including carrying basket and holding garments with left hand

O:

Initial evaluation of client factors 7/05/12	Reassessment of client factors 8/31/12
Total Active Motion of the left wrist: 125° Total active motion of the left thumb: 110° Grip Strength Ⓡ 41# Grip strength Ⓛ 15# (37% of Ⓡ) Pinch not tested Min edema Ⓑ thumbs	Total active motion of the left wrist: 160° Total active motion of the left thumb: 130° Grip strength Ⓡ 41# Grip strength Ⓛ 22# Pinch not tested No edema

Client has participated in eight 45-minute sessions in outpatient hand clinic since admission on 7/05/12. AROM and PROM have been performed and taught to client, and home program has been modified as she progressed. Hot packs and paraffin were administered, and the client has purchased a home paraffin unit. Electrical stimulation has been used to elicit specific motion and facilitate strengthening of the flexor pollicis longus. A strengthening program has been added to the HEP, and client is able to demonstrate all exercises correctly. Client has received education on the structure and use of the hand, common features of CMC arthritis, ergonomics of the workstation, energy conservation, use of heat for pain relief, and adapted techniques for ADLs. Client reports understanding the education and has been given written material covering the same content.

A: Increase in grip strength of 7# shows good progress in strength needed to perform functional tasks. Thumb AROM is now WFL, and total wrist AROM has increased 35°, allowing client to perform most work and ADL tasks Ⓘ in ways that do not damage the joint. Change to an ergonomic keyboard and understanding and correct self-administration of HEP indicate good potential to continue improvement without continued OT services.

P: Results of reevaluation indicate no further need for OT services at this time. Client to follow the home program of heat, exercise, and adapted techniques. Client was advised to call hand clinic if questions arise.

Brad Beneficence, OTR/L, CHT

Transition Plans

A transition plan is developed and written whenever a client transfers within a service delivery system from one setting to another (AOTA, 2008a). This is the responsibility of the OT, but, as with other stages of treatment, the OTA can contribute to this process (AOTA, 2010c). The purpose of the transition plan is to provide client information to the new service providers to prevent any interruption in care. According to the *Guidelines for Documentation of Occupational Therapy* (AOTA, 2008a), a transition plan summarizes the client's current occupational status, specifies what service setting the client is leaving and what setting the client is entering, and states how and when the transition will occur. It also lists what follow-up or recommended services would benefit the client, such as continued therapy, specific equipment, or necessary modifications.

XYZ Early Intervention Program
Occupational Therapy Department
Transition Plan

Name: Kidd, Kari   **Date of birth**: 4/29/09   **Gender**: Female   **Record #**: 87654
Date of plan: 4/11/2012   **Expected transition date**: May, 2012
Precautions/contraindications: Seizure disorder

Occupational history: Kari experienced head and orthopedic injuries following a MVA at 9 days of age. Since that time, she has had multiple cranial, hip, and leg surgeries. She is currently under the management of a neurologist as well as an orthopedist. The mother carries out a home program daily, which is designed to stimulate development.

S: The mother reports that although Kari's seizures, multiple surgeries, and illnesses have slowed her development, the family is hopeful that Kari will progress more rapidly through her developmental milestones now that the surgeries are finished and the seizures are under control.

O: Child received her first occupational therapy screening in the hospital 1 week post injury. She received formal developmental assessments at 2, 4, 6, 12, and 24 months of age. Parents were instructed in a home program following the initial formal assessment. Regular OT treatment sessions were started at 12 months of age and have continued to this date. Child has been seen twice weekly in her home and monthly in the Birth-to-Three clinic. She is now eligible for preschool services as she is turning 3.

    Current occupational performance: Current problems being treated in occupational therapy include visual regard and visually directed reach, midline orientation, postural symmetry, and motor overflow. Current goals for Kari include functional reach, grasp and release, rolling, and ability to sustain anti-gravity positions for ADLs and developmental play activities.

A: At 3 years of age, Kari is at about a 4-month level of development. Although the mother provides a stimulating environment, Kari would benefit from continuation of regular occupational therapy, physical therapy, and speech therapy services to facilitate her continued progress through the developmental sequence.

P: Kari will receive her first preschool service evaluation next month in May of 2012. Parents have been instructed in a home program, which has been updated as child has progressed in treatment. Home program will continue through the transition to Preschool Services.

Alice Altruism, OTR/L

Discharge Report

When therapy is no longer necessary in a particular setting, a discharge report (also called a discontinuation report) is written. It provides a synopsis of the client's changes or progress from start of care to the present time regarding ability to engage in occupation. Discharge reports are the responsibility of the OT, but the therapist can delegate parts of this process to the OTA as appropriate (AOTA, 2010c). Discharge notes often follow a specific format. Content should include the date and purpose of the referral; a summary of the client's condition; a comparison of initial evaluation findings to status at time of discharge; and a summary of course of treatment, such as types of interventions/programs, physical agent modalities, splints, assistive devices, modification of the task or environment, and client/caregiver education. Discharge reports also summarize progress and outcomes relating to occupational performance and specify any recommendations for follow-up care (AOTA, 2008a). Recommendations may include continued therapy in a different setting, home exercise programs, specialized equipment or durable medical equipment, home or workplace modifications, support groups, or community services. The number of OT sessions provided may also be listed in the discharge report. Discharge reports may be written in a SOAP or narrative format, or the facility may have a special form that is used. Some facilities use the same (or similar) form for evaluation, reevaluation, and discharge, making it easier to prepare the discontinuation report.

There are many reasons that an occupational therapy client is discharged or treatment is discontinued. It is important for the discharge report to indicate the circumstances or reasons for discharge. Table 16-2 lists possible reasons for discontinuing occupational therapy.

Table 16-2
Reasons for Discharge

- Occupational therapy outcomes were met
- Client discharged from facility or agency
- No further occupational therapy is necessary
- Duplication of services
- Client not making progress
- Client became ill/was hospitalized
- MD discontinued therapy
- Reimbursement issues/managed care
- Client requires more specialized services than can be provided at this facility
- Client noncompliant or refusing therapy
- Poor attendance
- Client expired
- Client moved
- Client decided to receive services elsewhere

The following is an example of a discharge report using the SOAP format:

Rosy Rehabilitation Center
Occupational Therapy Department
Discharge Report

Name: Doe, Jane   **Record #**: 246810   **DOB**: 11/10/38
Dx: ⓇTHR   **Date of surgery**: 9/21/12   **Admission date**: 9/25/12
Date: 10/19/12   **Time**: 3:00 PM   **Gender**: F

S: Client reports that she is very pleased with the outcome of her occupational therapy treatment, and with her ability to take care of herself at home. She reports no steps to the front entrance of a one-story home, and no architectural barriers inside the house. She reports owning the following adaptive equipment: wheeled walker, reacher, dressing stick, sock aid, long shoehorn, tub bench, raised toilet seat, and grab bars around the toilet and tub area.

O: Client participated in OT bedside and in clinic area 20/20 sessions from SOC on 9/25/12

ADL status on 9/25/12	ADL status on 10/19/12
Mod Ⓐ in transfers	SBA in transfers
Mod Ⓐ in toileting	Ⓘ in toileting
Mod Ⓐ in feeding	SBA in feeding after set-up
Mod Ⓐ in dressing	Dressing from arm chair requires set-up only, but SBA for standing and pulling pants up over hips
Max Ⓐ for safety in bathing	SBA in bathing with min Ⓐ w/c ↔ shower using tub bench

Client education in adaptive techniques and HEP were discussed with client, and client demonstrated ability to perform correctly and adhere to all total hip precautions. Home modifications discussed with client and caregiver.

A: Client has made good progress in self-care activities as shown by differences in admitting and discharge abilities. Because caregiver is available to provide SBA needed for safety in ADL tasks, all treatment goals have been met, and client is ready for discontinuation of occupational therapy services.

P: Client to continue home exercise program. Adaptive equipment recommended: walker basket and reacher holder for walker. Client to continue outpatient PT. No direct OT services recommended at this time.

Patty Patience, OTR/L

Now here is the same information using a narrative format:

Rosy Rehabilitation Center
Occupational Therapy Department
Discharge Note

Name: Doe, Jane   **Record #**: 246810   **DOB**: 11/10/38
Dx: ⓇTHR   **Date of surgery**: 9/21/12
Gender: F   **Admission date**: 9/25/12
Date: 10/19/12   **Time**: 3:00 PM

Course of Rehabilitation: Client participated in 20/20 sessions from SOC on 9/25/12. Skilled instruction in adaptive techniques for ADLs provided. Client's progress was good, and she demonstrated ability to adhere to total hip precautions. All treatment goals met. Client now requires SBA in all transfers, lower body ADLs, upper body ADLs, grooming/hygiene. She is able to complete toileting Ⓘ. Client also requires SBA in feeding. Following set-up, client is able to perform dressing seated in armchair and using wheeled walker, but she needs SBA for standing and to pull pants up over hips. Client needs min Ⓐ w/c ↔ shower using tub bench but is able to complete bathing with SBA.

Client Education: Recommendations for additional adaptive equipment and modifications to home discussed with client and caregiver. Client and caregiver were instructed in home exercise program of exercise bands, free weights, wands, and other activities to choose from for Ⓑ UE strengthening. HEP discussed with client and client demonstrated ability to perform exercises correctly.

Discharge Recommendations/Referrals: Discharge with home caregiver. Continue home exercise program. Adaptive equipment recommended: walker basket and reacher holder for walker. Client already has wheeled walker, reacher, dressing stick, sock aid, long shoehorn, and functional bathroom equipment and has demonstrated ability to use these correctly and safely. Client will continue outpatient PT. No direct OT services are recommended at this time.

Patty Patience, OTR/L

Chapter 17

Documentation in Different Practice Settings

This chapter will look at documentation for different practice settings, each of which has some requirements specific to the setting or the primary source of payment. Documentation for these situations is different in some ways from the examples you have learned so far. Realize that the present requirements are always subject to change based on federal and state regulations, payer requirements, or changes in clinical practice guidelines.

Documentation in Mental Health

If you go from a job in a rehabilitation center to one in a mental health (or behavioral health) setting, you might think that nothing you have learned about documentation applies. Some of the language used in mental health settings may appear more subjective and general than what you have learned already. Documentation and treatment will reflect different criteria and terminology regarding performance skills, client factors, goals, and interventions as compared to those typically assessed or addressed in physical rehabilitation settings. Also, a multidisciplinary approach is often used in mental health settings to establish problems, goals, and interventions. Occupational therapy is often regarded as part of a broader treatment service designated as adjunctive therapy, expressive therapy, or activity therapy; disciplines that fall under this umbrella include therapeutic recreation specialists, music therapists, art therapists, and dance therapists. Professional roles often overlap and there is a blurring of professional identities. Intervention is often provided in groups or as part of a therapeutic environment or milieu. Reimbursement may not be discipline specific and therapy services may be included in the comprehensive daily rate for the facility. For example, clients with Medicare who receive inpatient psychiatric hospital services come under the Prospective Payment System, which pays a federal per-diem rate (CMS, 2012f). Thus, any occupational therapy services provided in those circumstances are not billed separately. However, outpatient occupational therapy is a separate covered service when provided through a partial hospitalization program where the rules for Medicare Part B apply (CMS, 2012f).

Occupational therapy practitioners have traditionally considered the holistic needs of those who receive our services. OTs and OTAs look at the physical, cognitive, social, emotional, and contextual factors that affect role performance and quality of life (AOTA, 2008b, 2008c). OTs and OTAs intervene to promote psychosocial well being and to facilitate engagement in desired life activities across all practice areas. Our clients in behavioral/mental health settings have significant psychosocial problems that create serious disruptions in their ability to take part in meaningful occupations. Occupational therapy practitioners in this practice area have a "toolbox" of psychosocial interventions that are a viable and fundamental component of occupational therapy practice.

Morreale MJ, Borcherding S.
The OTA's Guide to Documentation:
Writing SOAP Notes, Third Edition (pp 165-178).
© 2013 SLACK Incorporated.

Evaluation Reports and Intervention Plans

Initial evaluation reports may be performed by the OT (with contributions from the OTA). However, evaluation reports are often, instead, a collaborative effort involving all of the disciplines included in activity therapy, thereby losing some of the individual professional identity of occupational therapy. Third-party payers often require that facilities bundle therapy into the daily rate rather than billing individual therapies separately. Having an integrated "activities" or adjunctive therapy department is usually more cost effective than having a separate occupational therapy department. Even so, occupational therapy practitioners should consider an occupational profile essential in order to plan appropriate and effective interventions as the *Framework-II* suggests (AOTA, 2008b). Mental illness, poor coping mechanisms, or the misuse of alcohol or drugs all impact quality of life and the ability to engage in meaningful occupations. The OT, with assistance from the OTA, looks at the areas of occupation that are disrupted by the client's condition, the dysfunctional behaviors manifested by the illness or disorder, the influencing contextual factors, available supports, and the client's goals. The occupational therapy practitioners use this information to contribute to the treatment team's multidisciplinary problem list and intervention plan.

The "therapeutic milieu," or the setting's total environment, is often considered essential in caring for clients who have mental conditions. Ideally, each discipline assesses the client's needs and strengths, and then the team meets to formulate and prioritize a list of the client's problems. Problems in a mental health (or behavioral health) practice setting are traditionally divided into two parts. First, the problem itself is stated in one or two words, such as *"chemical dependence," "noncompliant behavior,"* or *"suicide risk."* Next, a description of the behavioral manifestations indicates the areas of occupation and underlying limiting factors involved.

> **Problem**: Suicide risk
> **Behavioral manifestations**: During the week prior to admission, the client verbalized suicidal ideation, stating that life was no longer worth living. On the day of admission, he had purchased a handgun.
>
> **Problem**: Chemical dependence
> **Behavioral manifestations**: Mark has been using alcohol since age 12 with increasing frequency over the last year, and also admits to using cocaine, "crystal," opium, and marijuana, resulting in a failed marriage, loss of two jobs, and involvement with the criminal justice system.
>
> **Problem**: Noncompliant behavior
> **Behavioral manifestations**: Client disobeys foster parents by running away, refusing to follow rules or requests, and engaging in sexual activity, resulting in six foster home placements in the past 4 years.

From this problem list, each individual discipline suggests goals, objectives, and treatment interventions appropriate to that discipline. In community mental health settings, occupational therapy goals can be related more easily and clearly to areas of occupational engagement. An **individualized treatment plan** (ITP) is developed, which is a contract for change between the client and the treatment team. Major concerns or problems identified in the evaluation are documented on the ITP, and each discipline's goals, objectives, and interventions are written into one comprehensive plan. The client collaborates in the intervention process and signs the treatment plan to demonstrate agreement with it. Similar types of plans are developed by teams in schools and rehabilitation settings, but mental health plans differ in that all team members work toward the same goals through different interventions. At some facilities, goals and objectives are selected from computer programs or provided on preprinted sheets for the problems most commonly treated, as illustrated later in this chapter. Because of short length of stay, a client may even be discharged before a comprehensive treatment plan can be formalized or all goals can be addressed.

In order for multidisciplinary treatment plans to be successful, the client (and family or significant other, if they are a part of the client's present life) must be actively involved. Each member of the treatment team must be willing to cooperate in a coordinated effort to effect change. In addition, the plan must be periodically reviewed to assess its effectiveness and to change or modify any interventions that have not been effective.

Intervention Strategies

OTs and OTAs use communication skills, empathy, and therapeutic use of self as part of the occupational therapy process to establish client relationships, identify meaningful occupations, and determine barriers to occupational performance (Kannenberg & Greene, 2003). A variety of interventions are used in mental health to promote empowerment, facilitate a positive self-concept, and enable personal change. Occupational therapy interventions are directed toward helping the client develop or remediate specific life skills for occupational roles within the home, workplace, community, and other contexts. OTs and OTAs help clients create an action plan for wellness recovery and provide instruction and practice to develop and support healthy habits and routines, life decision-making skills, coping strategies (e.g., for stress, depression, anger), organizational skills, communication/interaction skills, etc. (AOTA, 2011).

Interventions may be specific to occupational therapy or may be broader and applicable to activity therapy. Often, the choice of interventions depends largely upon what treatment groups are being provided by the facility. Intervention strategies are implemented within the groups, creating an interesting challenge for the OTA to address each client's particular needs at the same time. For example, most clients may attend communication groups or craft/activity groups, but within those groups, you will customize the way you choose to improve communication skills or task behaviors for each individual client. With a little experience, you will learn to individualize goals effectively for each participant while still providing for the needs of the group as a whole.

When planning intervention strategies, the treatment team considers the client's assets (e.g., intelligence, good verbal skills, self-awareness, etc.) as important tools that the client will use in overcoming problems. A "strength" in this context is an ability, a skill, or an interest that the client has used in the past or has the potential for using. Assets can include such things as the client's interests (e.g., enjoys playing music, gardening, knitting); abilities (e.g., writes well, accepts personal responsibility, is well organized); relationship skills (e.g., has a good relationship with spouse or adult children); and social support systems (e.g., AA group, clergy keeps in contact). Assets may also be past abilities that the treatment team wants to encourage as treatment progresses (e.g., Client was physically active before she became ill). Some interests (e.g., enjoys going to bars or casinos on weekends) may not be assets.

Ideally, occupational therapy documentation in psychosocial programs should be objective, measurable, realistic, and reflective of the occupation base of our profession. This means that your documentation must center on the client's occupational profile and the client's ability to engage in necessary and valued life activities and roles.

Contact and Progress Notes

The use of contact notes and progress notes vary by facility and funding source. If a client with Medicare has a mental health diagnosis and is seen in home health, the Medicare standards for home health apply. In a situation where progress notes rather than treatment notes are used, the occupational therapy practitioner keeps a log of attendance and might jot down informal notations about participation and behaviors that show progress each day. Although these may not be structured or formal entries into the record, they may be used later to compile a progress note in the health record at regular intervals.

When you begin thinking in the language of mental health, terms like *brightened affect*, *less delusional*, *improved mood*, or *increased self-esteem* begin to enter your vocabulary, and you may be tempted to write in less objective and measurable terms. However, there are definite observable behaviors that can help you determine that the client's affect is brighter or mood is improved. Perhaps you are seeing the client attend occupational therapy group with makeup applied or hair combed, initiate conversation three times in a group session, smile twice in 15 minutes, or respond to your "good morning" by making eye contact. Perhaps the client needs less time to get up and dress in the morning, is more easily persuaded to attend occupational therapy, or is able to select and carefully complete a craft project without verbal prompting. All of these indicators are measurable, and it is very helpful to the treatment team if you are able to report your skilled observations in measurable and behavioral terms.

Managed care, along with the trend toward role diffusion, is making it more difficult to document occupational therapy as a service that offers good value for the dollars spent in mental health care. You, as an OTA, need to focus on documenting functional changes that are cost effective and meaningful to both the payer and to the consumer. Individuals with serious mental illness or chemical dependency often have a myriad of factors that hinder their ability to engage in meaningful occupation. OTs and OTAs working in mental health settings need to communicate clearly how our unique services impact the client's ability to appropriately engage in pertinent occupations and achieve "successful, meaningful, and lasting functional outcomes" (Kannenberg and Greene, 2003 p. CE-1).

Critical Care Pathways in Mental Health

As length of stay has become shorter for psychiatric diagnoses, some mental health/behavioral health settings use critical care pathways and computer-generated intervention plans for the most common problems seen in that setting. These methods save time and can be customized to the client by adding desired outcomes and treatment interventions tailored to the individual's needs. Critical care pathways in mental health are multidisciplinary and are conceptually the same as those in rehabilitation. The plan for the client's care is preplanned for each day and for each discipline. This makes the most efficient use of staff time during the client's short length of stay while still making sure the client's needs are met.

Computer-Generated Plans

In an electronic "mix-and-match" program, the computer provides prompts from which the team or the individual clinician selects the problem statements, goals, objectives, and treatment interventions or methods that will be used for the individual consumer. Usually, the problems are expressed briefly in these prepackaged treatment planning sheets, such as "*depressed mood*," "*drug abuse*," or "*suicide risk*." Then, the client's specific behavioral manifestations are written in.

The treatment team chooses the client's goals from a menu of long-term goals, or **outcomes**, such as the following:

Client will report the absence of suicidal ideation.

or

Client will identify three new coping strategies to use when he feels the urge to use drugs.

During the client's hospitalization, all members of the multidisciplinary treatment team work on the selected goals. On a computer-generated form, there is also a list of potential interventions that would also be selected and addressed by the treatment team. Interventions on this menu might include such strategies as the following:

- Evaluate the client.
- Encourage the client to express emotions.
- Teach new coping skills.
- Encourage the client to verbalize alternatives to previous coping strategies.
- Assist the client to develop a discharge plan that will prevent recurrence.

Appropriate interventions are chosen for use with each client, and each discipline implements the interventions in its own way. Social work adapts interventions to individual and group therapy and nursing implements the interventions on the unit, but occupational therapy will implement the interventions in groups and in activities relating to occupational performance. In regard to the five intervention strategies listed previously, the OTA might do the following:

- Assist the OT in data collection for the occupational profile.
- Assist the OT in determining specific problems in each area of occupation.
- Use occupational therapy media to encourage the client to express emotions.
- Use occupational therapy groups to teach new coping skills and to help the client to find alternatives to strategies that have not worked well in the past.
- Provide feedback to the OT and client regarding task behaviors and performance skills as they relate to occupational performance.
- Help the client make a plan for any areas of occupation that were part of the previous problem.

In order to implement the multidisciplinary interventions, sheets are provided for each of the common goals. The interventions are individualized to the client by stating behavioral manifestations of the problem and by adding and deleting outcomes and/or interventions. The sheets also list the responsible staff member. This chapter includes an example of a prepackaged treatment planning sheet for alcohol dependence. It is provided only as a representation of what might be seen in clinical practice. Each setting will have its own protocols, but this will give you an idea of how a problem might be handled.

Let us consider another example: a female client admitted to a psychiatric unit following a suicide attempt. If the treatment team were using a computer-generated plan for this client, the first step would be to go to the computer and pull up some multidisciplinary treatment planning sheets. Some of the choices might be:

- Suicide attempt
- Anger
- Poor self-esteem

On each sheet, there would be a place to identify the client's behavior in relation to the problem.

Problem: Suicide attempt
Behavioral manifestations: During 2 days prior to admission, the client verbalized suicidal ideation, stating that her life was no longer worth living. On the day of admission, she took an overdose of sleeping pills and was brought to the ER by ambulance.

Problem: Anger
Behavioral manifestations: For the past 6 months, client has been fighting with her husband, resulting in marital separation, physical destruction of household objects, and high levels of stress.

Problem: Poor self-esteem
Behavioral manifestations: For the past month, client has shown diminished interest in her appearance, resulting in an unkempt look at home and work. She has been verbalizing self-deprecating statements regarding her looks, self-worth, and future plans.

Next follows a list of interventions commonly used for that problem, starting with evaluation and ending with discharge planning. Interventions on the list that do not apply to this client would be deleted, and any additional interventions unique to this client would be written in. The list of interventions would include some basic interventions such as, "*Encourage client to express emotions*" and "*Teach new coping skills,*" and other interventions would be added as appropriate for a particular situation such as, "*Encourage positive self-concept,*" "*Facilitate attention to grooming and personal hygiene,*" or "*Encourage interaction with peers.*" The groups provided by the facility would be listed as interventions, and the OT and OTA would plan for ways to make the daily occupational therapy groups meet the client's needs. There would be a list of desired outcomes for each client's identified problems, with a place to add outcomes specific to the situation.

Behavioral Health Multidisciplinary Treatment Plan

Client Name:
Problem #:
Behavioral manifestations:
Record #:
Problem name: Alcohol Dependence   **Date identified:**

Desired Outcomes	Target Date	Date Achieved
1. Client will verbally acknowledge that alcohol use has been a problem and will state an intent to abstain from alcohol use.		
2. Client will have developed at least three new ways to manage stress and will have demonstrated use of these.		
3. Client will have an aftercare plan in place.		
4. Client will have established a 5-day period of sobriety and of attending AA meetings daily.		
5.		
6.		

Treatment Interventions	Staff Responsible
1. Evaluate the client's alcohol intake and use patterns.	
2. Provide individual, group, and family therapy.	
3. Educate regarding the disease model of chemical dependency.	
4. Provide opportunities to express feelings.	
5. Teach coping skills.	
6. Assist client to restructure environmental situations.	
7. Evaluate and teach relationship skills.	
8. Facilitate peer confrontation and feedback.	
9. Introduce social/leisure activities that do not include alcohol.	
10.	
11.	

I agree with this plan.

_____
Client's signature

Documentation in School-Based Practice

Occupational therapy practitioners working in the public school system use concepts and language that are unique to that setting. Therefore, documentation in school settings is different from the notes occupational therapy practitioners might write in other practice areas. The children with disabilities in your school caseload will each have an intervention plan called an **Individualized Education Program** (IEP). This IEP consists of strengths, weaknesses, goals, and interventions that are **educationally based**; that is, focused on behaviors and skills the student needs to be successful in school. The IEP is a formal, multidisciplinary written plan. It is established at an annual meeting for each child classified as needing special services. The plan is compiled by therapists, teachers, and parents, plus any other appropriate professionals involved with the child (such as a psychologist, blind mobility specialist, sign language interpreter, social worker, or special educator). As each child's needs are different, not all students with an IEP require occupational therapy services.

In 2004, President George W. Bush reauthorized the Individuals with Disabilities Education Act (IDEA), with the majority of the new law effective July 2005 (U.S. Department of Education, 2006). The regulations revised and outlined the following requirements for general content of an IEP:

- A statement of the child's present levels of *academic achievement and functional performance*
- A statement of measurable, annual academic and functional goals designed to meet the child's needs (resulting from disability) to enable participation and progress in the general education curriculum and also meet other educational needs of the child
- A description of benchmarks or short-term objectives for children with disabilities who take alternate assessments aligned to meet special standards
- A description of how the child's progress toward meeting the annual goals will be measured and reported (such as reports at specific intervals or concurrent with the issuance of report cards)
- A statement of the special education and related services and supplementary aids and services (based on peer reviewed research to the extent practicable) to be provided to, or on behalf of, the child
- A statement of any individual appropriate accommodations that are necessary to measure the academic achievement and functional performance of the child on state- and district-wide assessments
- IEPs relating to transition services must include appropriate, measurable postsecondary goals based upon age-appropriate transition assessments (related to training, education, employment, and, where appropriate, independent living skills) along with the transition services needed to assist the child in reaching those goals

Adapted from U.S. Department of Education. (2006). Individualized Education Program (IEP). Retrieved from http://idea.ed.gov/explore/view/p/%2Croot%2CTopicalBrief%2C10%2C

Model forms were established by the Department of Education to help schools meet the IDEA requirements (U.S. Dept. of Education, n.d.). In a school setting, the OT is responsible for directing the occupational therapy evaluation, establishing the occupational therapy component of the IEP, and implementing or overseeing occupational therapy treatment. The OTA might provide feedback throughout this process by implementing delegated assessments and interventions. The IEP is truly a shared effort. Based on each discipline's role and assessment, the IEP for each child details current educational status, strengths, weaknesses, goals, and interventions for the current school year. As the treatment principles, concepts, and outcomes for the entire team are collaborative, there may or may not be a distinct list of occupational therapy goals per se. However, the OT and OTA can play important roles in helping the child succeed in meeting curriculum standards and outcomes established by the district or team. Even though the child might have a particular medical condition or deficits in other areas of life, the IEP and interventions focus on the child's skills that need to be mastered in the educational setting. A student's weaknesses in school may include a number of areas such, as the following:

- Classroom behaviors and skills (attention to task, handwriting, scissors use, copying from blackboard, organizational skills, sitting at desk, etc.)
- Academic achievement
- Personal and toilet hygiene (washing hands, feminine hygiene, managing clothing)
- Dressing (putting on coat or boots, changing for gym)
- Feeding (opening food containers/wrappers, managing finger foods or utensils, carrying meal tray)
- Ability to participate in extracurricular activities (drama, music, clubs, sports)

- Ability to manage the activity demands for various school contexts (cafeteria, gym, recess, locker room, library, school bus)
- Ability to navigate around the school (mobility, managing backpack, locker use, temporal considerations, etc.)
- Ability to relate effectively to staff and peers

It is also important to realize that, although a child may struggle academically in areas such as spelling, math, general knowledge, etc. due to a learning disability or cognitive impairment, occupational therapy may not be indicated in every case. Occupational therapy supports academic goals by addressing related underlying skills needed in the educational setting. The team determines what services are appropriate to best meet the needs of a particular child and occupational therapy may or may not be part of the plan.

Goal statements in the IEP are normally called *annual goals*, which are written for the duration of the school year, rather than using a timeline for each goal. **Benchmarks** or **objectives** are established to determine or grade the child's progress toward meeting his or her goals. As noted previously in the Department of Education regulations, the student's progress might be assessed quarterly along with the academic report cards or per other established intervals. In a school setting, it is important to set goals for specific educational components rather than underlying factors. Goals should be clearly written and defined so that the child's specific expected behavior or criterion can be observed and measured by others (Clark, 2005). These criteria can include specific district or state curriculum standards, grade level requirements, developmental milestones, professional judgment, peer performance, and parent or teacher expected outcomes (Clark, 2005). School districts may vary in how the frequency and duration of occupational therapy sessions are delineated in the IEP. The IEP might specify a particular number of sessions weekly or monthly (e.g., two times a week for 30 minutes each or once monthly for 45 minutes), or instead may just specify the total number of minutes that will be provided by the end of the school year. A sum total in the IEP allows for flexibility week to week according to the child's needs and the occupational therapy practitioner's discretion.

IEPs can be quite lengthy. The one provided in this chapter has been condensed to show aspects that are representative or most pertinent to occupational therapy.

Individualized Education Program

Name: Truman T.   **Date of Birth**: 7/24/2005   **Age**: 5 yrs, 11 mos
School Year: 2011-2012   **Grade Level**: Kindergarten
IEP Meeting Date: 7/22/2011   **IEP Initiation/Duration Dates**: 8/8/11 to 5/26/12

Present Level of Academic Achievement and Functional Performance: Truman will be six years old in just a few days. He was diagnosed with Pervasive Developmental Disorder (PDD) at age two. He attended the Early Childhood Special Education program for two years during the 2008-2009 and 2009-2010 school years and Kindergarten during the 2010-2011 school year. The decision has been made by the IEP team to retain Truman in Kindergarten for the upcoming 2011-2012 school year. Truman's parents are in agreement with this decision and hope that another year in Kindergarten will allow him to improve his academic performance and social skills prior to advancing to 1st grade. Truman does not qualify for Extended School Year services at this time. Truman spends the majority of his day in the general education classroom with a paraprofessional present for support with classroom participation. He spends 60 minutes daily in the special education classroom for additional 1:1 and small group instruction in reading and writing skills. He also participates in adaptive physical education twice weekly for 45 minutes.

Truman's verbal skills are delayed in comparison to same-age peers, although he has demonstrated considerable improvement over the past year. He is now able to communicate in three- to five-word sentences consistently. He also utilizes a Picture Exchange Communication System (PECS) to supplement his verbal communication.

Truman is easily distracted by auditory and visual stimuli in and near the classroom and has difficulty remaining in his seat for more than 5 minutes at a time. He has difficulty with transitions between activities and locations, but this has improved following implementation of a visual schedule. Truman sometimes responds with negative behaviors (yelling, hitting, pinching) when classmates inadvertently touch or bump into him during classroom activities.

Truman is hesitant to engage in play activities with his peers. He prefers to play alone and does not initiate interactions with peers. Toward the end of last school year, he was beginning to participate in some simple ball activities with others during recess with significant support from his paraprofessional. He will continue participation in a weekly after-school peer communication group led by the elementary school counselor.

(continued)

Truman is able to recognize all letters of the alphabet, but he does not yet read any words. He can copy the letters of his name when provided with a visual model, but legibility is inconsistent. His ability to copy other letters of the alphabet remains very inconsistent. Truman has difficulty achieving a tripod grasp on writing utensils and staying on the lines of standard writing paper. He also has difficulty with consistent letter size and spacing. His writing performance improves with the use of adaptive writing paper and rubber pencil grip. He does consistently copy basic shapes including circle, square, triangle, and cross.

Truman requires assistance to obtain and carry his tray in the lunchroom. He is easily upset by the noise in the lunchroom and often needs to be taken to a quieter room to finish lunch. Truman consistently indicates when he needs to use the restroom, but continues to have difficulty managing the button and zipper on his jeans. He needs hand-over-hand assistance to complete hand washing because he prefers to play in the water. Truman is now able to take his coat on and off independently. He can also manage Velcro tennis shoes independently.

Type of Service	Anticipated Frequency	Amount of Time	Location of Service
Special Education: Special education teacher will provide intensive reading and writing instruction in both 1:1 and small group formats.	Daily	60 minutes	Special Education Classroom
Supplementary Aids & Services: Truman will have a paraprofessional present throughout the school day except when with the special education teacher.	Daily	340 minutes	General Education Classroom & Across Settings
Program Modifications: Adaptive P.E.	Weekly	90 minutes	Indoor/Outdoor P.E. Settings
Accommodations for Assessments: Truman will be allowed additional time for completion of classroom and state assessments.	Weekly	60 minutes	General and Special Education Classrooms
Related Services: Occupational Therapy	Weekly	30 minutes	General and Special Education Classrooms & Across Settings
Related Services: Speech Language Pathology	Weekly	90 minutes	General and Special Education Classrooms & Across Settings

Annual Goal #1: Using compensatory strategies, Truman will demonstrate legible handwriting in the classroom with appropriate baseline orientation, letter size, and spacing with 80% accuracy on 4 of 5 consecutive days.

Evaluation Methods:
☐ Curriculum-Based Assessment
☐ State Assessments
☑ Data Collection Chart
☑ Work Samples
☐ Other:

Primary Implementers:
☑ General Education Teacher
☑ Special Education Teacher
☐ Physical Therapy
☑ Occupational Therapy
☐ Speech Language Pathology
☐ Other:

Measurable Benchmarks/Objectives:
1. Truman will demonstrate tripod grasp on writing utensils using adaptive pencil grip with 80% accuracy on 4 of 5 consecutive days.
2. Truman will write his first name on adaptive paper without a visual model, demonstrating appropriate letter formation, size, and line orientation on 4 of 5 consecutive days.
3. Truman will copy 22/26 lowercase letters onto adaptive paper using a visual model, demonstrating appropriate letter formation, size, and line orientation on 4 of 5 consecutive days.

Date of Mastery:
1.
2.
3.

(continued)

Annual Goal #2: Truman will demonstrate improved attention and work behaviors during classroom activities with no more than three sensory breaks per hour throughout the day on 4 of 5 consecutive days.

Evaluation Methods:	Primary Implementers:
☐ Curriculum-Based Assessment	☑ General Education Teacher
☐ State Assessments	☑ Special Education Teacher
☑ Data Collection Chart	☐ Physical Therapy
☐ Work Samples	☑ Occupational Therapy
☐ Other:	☐ Speech Language Pathology
	☐ Other:

Measurable Benchmarks/Objectives:	Date of Mastery:
1. Truman will remain seated at his desk or during circle time for 15 minutes with minimal verbal cues and no more than one sensory break.	1.
2. Truman will transition between classroom activities with minimal verbal cues using a visual schedule and without demonstrating negative behaviors (yelling, hitting, etc.) toward peers and staff with 80% accuracy on 4 of 5 consecutive days.	2.
3. Truman will tolerate unexpected touch from classmates without demonstrating negative behaviors (yelling, hitting, etc.) with 80% accuracy on 4 of 5 consecutive days.	3.

Annual Goal #3: Truman will demonstrate school-related self-care skills with no more than minimal assistance using adaptive strategies with 80% accuracy on 4 of 5 consecutive days.

Evaluation Methods:	Primary Implementers:
☐ Curriculum-Based Assessment	☐ General Education Teacher
☐ State Assessments	☐ Special Education Teacher
☑ Data Collection Chart	☐ Physical Therapy
☐ Work Samples	☑ Occupational Therapy
☐ Other:	☐ Speech Language Pathology
	☑ Other: Paraprofessional

Measurable Benchmarks/Objectives:	Date of Mastery:
1. Truman will complete toileting without assistance to manage clothing fasteners with 80% accuracy on 4 of 5 consecutive days.	1.
2. Truman will wash hands following a visual schedule with minimal verbal cues with 80% accuracy on 4 of 5 consecutive days.	2.
3. Truman will obtain/transport his lunch tray and remain seated in the cafeteria for the duration of the lunch period with minimal verbal cues on 4 of 5 consecutive days.	3.

Reprinted with permission from Gateley, C.A., & Borcherding, S. (2012). *Documentation manual for occupational therapy: Writing SOAP notes* (3rd ed.). Thorofare, NJ: SLACK Incorporated.

Skilled Nursing Facilities and Long-Term Care Settings

Medicare and Medicaid are primary funding sources for clients who receive subacute rehabilitation services in skilled nursing facilities. Therefore, occupational therapy documentation must reflect the need for skilled services, including the potential for functional change, to address pertinent safety concerns, or to prevent secondary medical complications. Documentation and interventions will normally focus on client factors and performance skills needed for the client to return home or function in other contexts, such as improving activity tolerance, safe functional mobility, or ADLs. Occupational therapy practitioners might recommend, fabricate, or modify items such as adaptive equipment, splints, positioning devices, or wheelchairs or implement other pertinent interventions. Clients sometimes participate in occupational therapy groups that address particular occupational performance skills or client factors such as a cooking group or an UE exercise group. In long-term care settings, clients with Medicare or Medicaid may also receive occupational therapy services if skilled rehabilitation is warranted. In those cases, the OT will address pertinent problem areas identified in the care plan in order to improve functional performance and quality of life (CMS, 2012c).

When a client with Medicare or Medicaid is admitted to a skilled nursing facility, the federally mandated Resident Assessment Instrument (RAI) is used to determine the level of care needed (CMS, 2012e). The assessment tool used in the RAI is called the *Minimum Data Set* (MDS) (CMS, 2012d). The MDS is a quality measure that considers all aspects of the client such as mood, behavior, mobility, ADL status, bowel and bladder function, nutrition, pain, skin integrity, etc. The MDS helps to identify a client's problem areas (called *care area triggers*) for which the treatment team can develop a plan of care (CMS, 2012d). The MDS is also used to monitor the overall quality of care in nursing homes and to provide consumers with access to information about all Medicare and Medicaid certified nursing homes in the United States (CMS, 2012e). You can view the MDS form and instructions on how to complete it at the CMS Web site (www.cms.gov/CMSForms).

Each discipline may be assigned a specific part of the MDS to complete in order to improve efficiency, team communication, and to facilitate a more holistic approach to care of the resident (CMS, 2012c, 2012e). Facilities may vary in how ADL, cognitive, or other sections are divided between occupational therapy, nursing, or other disciplines. Clients are then divided into Resource Utilization Groupings as part of the Prospective Payment System according to how much care they need (CMS, 2012e). This determines the reimbursement that the facility will receive based on the category or level of skilled services required. To substantiate this level of care, rehabilitation professionals typically document the exact number of therapy minutes provided for each individual client along with documenting the skilled intervention provided and the client's progress. If this entire process is not implemented or documented properly, the client will be unable to get the level of care needed. Also, inaccurate assessments or unrealistic predictions about rehabilitation potential may result in reimbursement problems for care rendered.

Specific formats and timelines for occupational therapy documentation will depend on the requirements of the particular facility, accrediting agency, and funding source such as Medicare or private insurance. Clients referred to occupational therapy will generally go through the occupational therapy evaluation process as described in Chapter 14. If the MDS is required, it does not take the place of a "regular" occupational therapy evaluation form or procedure. Subsequent intervention sessions may be documented by the OT as a progress report written at regular intervals (e.g., weekly or every 2 weeks), but the OTA can document or contribute information along the way. In addition, facilities or payers may require attendance logs, checklists, or contact notes for each client intervention or communication. The OTA involved with the client intervention or interaction will document what transpired using a SOAP note or other approved format, with cosignature of the OT if required. In accordance with facility and payer guidelines, the OT is responsible for reevaluation and transition reports as indicated and will also write a discharge or discontinuation report when the client leaves the facility or occupational therapy is no longer necessary.

Outpatient Documentation

Private Insurance and Managed Care

Documentation in outpatient settings depends on the requirements of the particular facility, accrediting agency, and payment source. Clients referred to outpatient occupational therapy will normally go through the evaluation process as described in Chapter 14. The occupational therapy department will typically have forms tailored to the particular practice area or specialization such as work hardening, cardiac or hand rehabilitation, low vision, sensory integration, etc. In addition to the facility form, if managed care is involved, that company might provide an additional form for the OT (or other team member/staff) to fill out delineating the client's problems, justification for skilled occupational therapy, and outlining the plan of care. The managed care company might only initially approve a set number of visits within a specific time frame. If additional therapy is warranted after those approved visits are completed, the therapist must make a formal request. This might require calling the case manager, sending a progress note or reevaluation report, or filling out another managed care form, in accordance with HIPAA and facility guidelines.

Depending on the facility and funding source, outpatient intervention sessions will usually be documented as progress notes at regular intervals, although attendance logs, checklists, or formal contact notes (e.g., SOAP note) might also be required for each visit. It is very important to document measurable, objective progress and any gains in specific functional abilities, as well as to indicate the limiting factors requiring continued occupational therapy.

The OTA involved with the client's intervention or communication will document what transpired, with cosignature of the OT when required. Your documentation and feedback as an OTA will provide important information to the OT, treatment team, and insurance company reviewers. Progress reports and reevaluation reports are written by the OT (with contributions from the OTA) according to facility guidelines and funding source. An occupational therapy discharge or discontinuation note is also written by the OT when the client leaves the facility or therapy is no longer necessary.

Medicare Documentation

For clients with Medicare B, current requirements for occupational therapy documentation are outlined in Chapter 15 of the *Medicare Benefit Policy Manual,* which can be found at the CMS Web site (www.cms.gov). In addition to delineating the criteria for contents of an initial evaluation, Medicare regulations clearly state the evaluation can only be performed and documented by the OT (CMS, 2008d, 2008e). Following evaluation, the OT establishes an intervention plan, which Medicare refers to as a *plan of care* (POC). The POC, at minimum, must include the client's diagnoses; the frequency, duration, type, and amount of occupational therapy services; occupational therapy long-term goals; professional signature with credentials; and the date (CMS, 2008b). Medicare also requires that this POC be **certified** (CMS, 2005a). A certified POC means that the client must be under the care of a physician (or approved non-physician provider [NPP]) who approves and signs the occupational therapy plan (CMS, 2005b, 2008c). This initial certification is good for 90 calendar days (from the initial treatment date) or for the duration delineated in the POC, whichever is less (CMS, 2008c). Once the POC is certified, any major changes to that plan (such as treating a different condition of that client or significantly changing the LTGs) requires documented written or verbal approval from the physician/NPP (CMS, 2008b). If a client is receiving multiple rehabilitation services, each discipline must develop a separate POC for certification (CMS, 2008b).

Periodic **progress reports** are required by Medicare at specified intervals and are written by the OT to justify that skilled therapy is still warranted (CMS, 2008d). Progress reports describe changes in the client's condition or the treatment provided along with the updating of goals; they may be written more frequently as needed, according to facility policy or the OT's professional judgment (CMS, 2008d). OTAs can document in the record and supplement information inbetween the OT's progress reports (CMS, 2008d). Formal **reevaluations** are implemented and documented by the OT at intervals determined by the OT's professional judgment or facility policy (CMS, 2008a, 2008d).

The purpose of **treatment notes**, according to Medicare guidelines, is to "create a record of all treatments and skilled interventions that are provided and to record the time of the services in order to justify the use of billing codes on the claim. Documentation is required for every treatment day, and every therapy service" (CMS, 2008d, p. 186). Medicare does not dictate the exact format of a treatment note but does require, at a minimum, the following content (CMS, 2008d):

- The date of treatment
- Each specific modality/intervention provided and billed
- Total timed code treatment minutes
- Total treatment time in minutes (only time that is billable)
- The qualified professional's signature and professional designation (who supervised or implemented the service)

If the occupational therapy supervisor did not actively communicate or participate in the session, it is not mandatory for the supervisor to cosign the OTA's note for clients with Medicare, although state regulations, practice acts, or facility policies might require that (CMS, 2008d). OTs and OTAs use clinical judgment to decide what additional information should be included in the treatment note regarding the client contact, such as client self-report, changes in status, reaction to intervention, etc. (CMS, 2008d). Review Chapter 3 for a description of Medicare's strict requirements for skilled occupational therapy and what is considered reasonable and necessary for the client's condition. The SOAP note guidelines throughout this manual will also help to ensure that your treatment notes will meet the criteria established by Medicare and other payers.

Acute Care

Occupational therapy practitioners working in acute care settings play a vital role, but they also face challenges such as short lengths of stay, medically fragile clients, and increased productivity demands due to cost-saving measures. Discharge planning begins the day the client is admitted and the treatment team provides intervention directed toward the client's needs for the expected discharge environment.

When an order for occupational therapy is received, the OT begins the evaluation process and establishes the intervention plan. Some facilities utilize clinical pathways for standard diagnoses such as total hip replacement or total knee replacement. Clinical pathways provide a daily blueprint for the designated care that should be provided by each discipline, including occupational therapy. In this case, there are preplanned interventions and goals for each day of the client's hospital stay, although those interventions can be modified according to the individual's needs. Occupational therapy priorities in acute care should reflect the client's occupational profile, medical needs, and expected roles and responsibilities upon discharge. As lengths of stay in acute care are usually brief, treatment will often focus on client/caregiver education, safety, activity tolerance, and basic functional tasks such as transfers, bed mobility, feeding, personal hygiene and grooming, upper body bathing, and dressing. Clients who have orthopedic, neurological, cardiopulmonary, or other conditions might also require various preparatory interventions such as therapeutic exercise programs, positioning, wound care, edema management, or splinting, all directed toward the goal of occupational engagement. OTs and OTAs may also recommend durable medical equipment, adaptive devices, modifications, or other supports that will be needed by the client at home.

Due to the client's rapidly changing status in the acute care environment, contact notes are normally written by the OT or OTA after each occupational therapy session. This will communicate important information to the treatment team about any changes in the client's condition, safety, activity tolerance, functional abilities, and barriers to occupational performance. Because of short lengths of stay, formal reevaluation reports are often not necessary. If the client is transferred to another service delivery setting within the organization, a transition plan is written; otherwise, a discharge or discontinuation note is written when the client is discharged from the facility or occupational therapy is no longer needed.

Home Care

Occupational therapy practitioners in home care work with people of all ages who are considered homebound; that is, the client would have severe difficulty receiving services outside of the home (CMS, 2003a). The client's residence could be a personal dwelling, relative's home, assisted living facility, or another noninstitutional place that the client considers to be his or her home (CMS, 2003b). Federal regulations mandate the gathering of specific outcomes data for nonmaternity clients with Medicare or Medicaid who are 18 years of age or older and who receive **skilled** services at home (CMS, 2011c). The method used to collect the required data is called the *Outcome and Assessment Information Set* (OASIS) and the current version used is the OASIS-C (CMS, 2011c). You can view the OASIS and instructions for how to complete it at the CMS Web site (www.cms.gov/CMSForms/). The OASIS requirements do not apply to clients only receiving nonskilled services in the home such as personal care, homemaker, or chore services (CMS, 2011c). The OASIS is completed at the start of care, recertification periods, discharge, and client transfer to another facility. It addresses the holistic needs of the client such as living situation (safety, hazards), supports, medical status/systems review, ADLs, nutrition, mobility, physical functioning, sleep patterns, etc. (CMS, 2011c).

If nursing is involved in the case, the RN will complete the OASIS at the start of care, but then the subsequent assessments may be completed by the RN, OT, PT, or SLP/ST if involved in that client's care (CMS, 2011c). The need for skilled occupational therapy alone can establish eligibility for Medicaid home health therapy services for adults, but in order for a client with Medicare to receive occupational therapy home health benefits, the client must also receive another skilled service such as PT, SLP, or nursing (CMS, 2011c). Thus, for clients requiring home therapy without skilled nursing care, the OT cannot complete the initial OASIS for a client with Medicare but can for clients with Medicaid (CMS, 2011c).

The physician must sign and approve (certify) the POC for all skilled services the client with Medicare will receive (CMS, 2003c). The OASIS does not take the place of a "regular" occupational therapy evaluation. The OT assesses the client's function and establishes a specific intervention plan directed toward the skilled, reasonable, and necessary treatment the client requires in the home environment (CMS, 2003d, 2011a). OT interventions in home care aim to improve specific BADLs, IADLs, activity tolerance, safety, functional mobility, and transfers and help prevent secondary medical complications (CMS, 2011a). In addition, occupational therapy interventions often include family/caregiver education and recommendations for adaptive equipment, safety, home modifications, or home exercise programs. Contact notes are typically written for each visit. Documentation requirements for Medicare include reassessments at specified intervals (CMS, 2011a). A discharge or discontinuation report is written when occupational therapy is no longer indicated. The Medicare requirements for occupational therapy are outlined in Chapter 7 of the *Medicare Benefit Policy Manual*, which can be found on the CMS Web site (www.cms.gov). Other funding sources will have different requirements.

Palliative Care

Occupational therapy practitioners who work in hospice or other practice settings where clients have terminal illnesses often provide palliative care rather than rehabilitation. Palliative care involves a philosophy of focusing on providing comfort, symptom relief, emotional support, and quality of life as clients prepare for death. Third-party payers look at therapy services slightly differently in these situations. As there is no expectation that the client will make progress in physical functioning, goals often center around quality of life issues such as pain control and maintaining the ability to engage in meaningful occupations. Goals might include traditional intervention approaches such as energy conservation, adaptive equipment, positioning, and family/caregiver education. Sometimes nontraditional interventions are also used, including relaxation, active listening, and complementary and alternative therapies.

Different Formats for Notes

Facilities may use **checklists**, **flow sheets**, or other types of forms created by the facility instead of SOAP notes to save time. With these other formats, information might be categorized slightly differently than if you are writing a SOAP note. Forms are a popular way to record an initial assessment because they allow quite a lot of information to be communicated with minimal time spent writing. Narrative notes are not formally organized into sections the way SOAP notes are. **Narrative** notes may present any information in any order desired. However, good narrative notes will contain the same type of content in the same basic order. It just will not be delineated as separate SOAP categories and will instead consist of a paragraph format.

Some facilities use **D.A.P.** notes (Data, Assessment, Plan), which are an adaptation of the SOAP format. In D.A.P. notes, the "D" (data) section contains both the "S" and the "O" information. Other formats of notes include **B.I.R.P.**, **P.I.R.P.**, or **S.I.R.P.** notes. These types of notes are sometimes used in mental health practice settings with the information distributed as follows:

B: The **behavior** that is exhibited by the client
I: The treatment **intervention** provided by the OT or OTA
R: The client's **response** to the intervention provided
P: The therapist's **plan** for continued intervention, based on the client's response

P: The **problem/purpose** of the treatment
IRP for intervention, response and plan, as above

S: The **situation**
IRP for intervention, response, and plan, as above

In this chapter, you have learned that practice settings vary in their formats and requirements for documentation according to the funding source, facility policy, and state and federal guidelines. The next chapter will present additional examples of occupational therapy notes for different stages of treatment and various practice settings.

Worksheet 17-1
Types of Documentation

Match each of the types of documentation below to the descriptions that follow.

    A. Contact Note
    B. Minimum Data Set
    C. Initial Evaluation
    D. Discontinuation Report
    E. Transition Plan
    F. IEP
    G. OASIS
    H. Progress Report
    I. Reevaluation Report
    J. Intervention Plan
    K. Occupational Profile

1. _____ Outcome measure required by Medicare and Medicaid for use in home care

2. _____ Yearly multidisciplinary plan established for a particular student requiring special services

3. _____ Contains goals and specific treatment approaches relating to desired client outcomes

4. _____ Written when occupational therapy services are no longer needed

5. _____ Interdisciplinary assessment used in a skilled nursing facility to determine a client's problem areas and care plan

6. _____ Summarizes course of treatment and progress toward achieving goals during specified intervals

7. _____ Written following a treatment session and can include intervention provided, pertinent phone conversations, or meetings

8. _____ Consists of an occupational profile and factors affecting engagement in occupation

9. _____ A determination of the client's present status as compared to start of care, including progress, problems, and revision of goals

10. ___ Includes the client's roles, responsibilities, and factors such as values, culture, physical and social environments, age, and educational level

11. _____ Written to provide consistency when a client switches from one setting to another during the treatment continuum

Morreale, M. J., & Borcherding, S. (2013). *The OTA's guide to documentation: Writing SOAP notes (3rd ed.).* Thorofare, NJ: SLACK Incorporated.

Chapter 18

Examples of Different Kinds of Notes

This final chapter provides examples of notes from different stages of treatment and from a variety of practice settings. The first group of notes illustrates different stages of the intervention process, while the second set provides examples of single treatment sessions in different practice settings.

Examples of Notes for Different Stages of Treatment

Examples of Treatment Notes for Different Kinds of Treatment Sessions

Most of the notes in this section were written by students, faculty, and practicing therapists. The signatures, names, and other information have been modified or fabricated to make the notes anonymous. Also, all required demographic data may not be present on these examples, but they would be included in a "real" note.

Morreale MJ, Borcherding S.
The OTA's Guide to Documentation:
Writing SOAP Notes, Third Edition (pp 179-190).
© 2013 SLACK Incorporated.

Acute Care Hospital: Initial Evaluation Report

Name: Doe, Jane   **Age**: 80   **Primary Dx**: Ⓛ THR   **Secondary Dx**: Hypertension
Primary payment source: Medicare   **Secondary payment source**: none
Admission date: 9/2/12   **Date of referral**: 9/3/12   **Health Record #**: 34567
Estimated length of stay: 4 days   **Physician**: B. Paynefree, MD
History of present condition: Client reports that yesterday morning she went upstairs at home to use the bathroom because there was none on the first floor. She became lightheaded, fell down the stairs, and broke her hip. She was admitted for a total hip replacement yesterday.
Brief occupational profile: Client reports living alone and being Ⓘ in all ADLs prior to admission. Her husband died 3 years ago and her family lives out of town and cannot stay with her. She wants to return home. Client has supportive neighbors and lives in a small town where she is retired from her position as a second grade teacher. She lives in a townhouse across the street from the elementary school. She is in the habit of visiting with the children and some of their families when school is out each day. She is also active in church activities and belongs to the choir.

Date: 9/3/12   **Time**: 8:30 AM
Occupational Therapy Evaluation Report

S: Client stated that she would like to "get this leg well" and go home to "live a regular life."

O: Client participated in 45-minute evaluation in hospital room to assess BADL capabilities after Ⓛ THR. Client educated on use of ADL equipment for self-care tasks and adherence to hip precautions. Client demonstrated ability to repeat 2/4 precautions. During ADL evaluation, client was observed flexing 8° to 10° beyond 90° and required 4 verbal cues to remain at or below 90° during the 45-minute session. Other three hip precautions were followed Ⓘ. After set-up, client was able to complete sponge bath at sink for upper body and used dressing stick with washcloth and verbal cues for lower body. Client PWB Ⓛ LE and required min Ⓐ for balance with sit ↔ stand to bathe back peri area. Client able to complete upper body dressing after set-up and able to don underwear and pants over hips using a dressing stick. Client able to don socks using sock aid after set-up with min verbal cues. Client completed grooming tasks and oral care Ⓘ. Following min verbal cues, client demonstrated good problem solving by trying different body positions to perform ADLs while adhering to hip precautions and demonstrated understanding of adaptive aids by utilizing reacher and dressing stick correctly after instruction. Client demonstrated ↓ ADL tolerance as she required four 2-minute rest breaks during dressing tasks. Client then transported via w/c to OT clinic for 15-minute evaluation of client factors:
Ⓡ hand dominant
Ⓑ UE AROM: WFL   Ⓑ UE strength: WFL
Ⓑ UE sensation: intact   Grip strength Ⓡ 47#, Ⓛ 43#
Tripod pinch Ⓡ 10#, Ⓛ 5#   Lateral pinch Ⓡ 10#; Ⓛ 5#

A: Client demonstrated good motivation, problem-solving skills, and understanding of equipment use, all of which indicate excellent rehab potential. Upper body strength and AROM WFL are assets for learning adaptive self-care techniques and functional mobility. Although client is able to complete grooming tasks and oral care Ⓘ, decreased performance skills such as poor endurance, ↓ standing balance, and inconsistent compliance with hip precautions create safety concerns for lower body dressing and bathing. These problem areas negatively impact client's ability to be Ⓘ and safe in ADL tasks. Client would benefit from skilled instruction on hip precautions and use of adaptive equipment with ADL performance, and therapeutic activities that facilitate dynamic standing balance and ↑ ADL activity tolerance. Exploration of interim living arrangement or possible continued home visits and home equipment procurement will be needed if progress warrants discharge to home.

P: OT twice daily for 1 hour the next 3 days to ↑ Ⓘ in self-care tasks through instruction on hip precautions, use of adaptive equipment, and tasks to ↑ activity tolerance and dynamic standing balance.

LTG: By anticipated discharge on 9/7/12, client will:

1. Safely complete lower body dressing and bathing with modified Ⓘ utilizing adaptive equipment with 100% adherence to hip precautions.
2. Demonstrate safe toileting with modified Ⓘ using rolling walker and bedside commode.

STG:

1. By next treatment session, client will transfer SBA sit ↔ stand using bedside commode and rolling walker, and manage clothing with no more than 2 verbal cues.
2. By 2nd session, client will don shoes & socks 100% of time with modified Ⓘ, utilizing adaptive techniques & devices with 100% adherence to hip precautions.

3. By 3rd session, client will ↑ activity tolerance for ADLs as demonstrated by no more than one 30-second rest break during lower body dressing task of donning underwear and slacks with SBA.

4. By 4th session, client will perform toileting with SBA using commode frame over toilet, wheeled walker, and adhering to total hip precautions.

5. By 4th session, client will safely bathe her peri area with modified Ⓘ utilizing adaptive techniques and devices with 100% adherence to hip precautions.

Signature: *Kim Kindness, OTR/L*

Intervention Plan

Name: Doe, Jane   **Age**: 80   **Primary Dx**: Ⓛ THR   **Secondary Dx**: HTN

Strengths: UE strength & AROM WFL; intact cognition and motivation to return home

Functional Problem Statement #1: ↑ fatigue, decreased compliance with THR precautions, and low activity tolerance make client unsafe in ADL tasks.

LTG #1: By anticipated discharge on 9/7/12, client will safely complete lower body dressing and bathing with modified Ⓘ utilizing adaptive equipment with 100% adherence to hip precautions.

Short-Term Goals	Interventions
STG #1: By 2nd session, client will don shoes & socks 100% of time with modified Ⓘ utilizing adaptive techniques and devices with 100% adherence to hip precautions.	1. Instruct and have client verbalize 4/4 hip precautions. 2. Provide written handouts of hip precautions 3. Instruct in use of adaptive techniques and devices followed by demonstration of use in dressing activities.
STG #2: By 3rd session, client will ↑ activity tolerance for ADLs as demonstrated by no more than one 30-second rest break during dressing task of donning underwear and slacks with SBA.	1. Educate client and provide written instructions on energy conservation techniques. Evaluate understanding by her application during ADL tasks; ask about how she performs ADL tasks at home. 2. Continue instruction in use of adaptive techniques/devices followed by demonstration of use in dressing activities. 3. Instruct in manipulation of clothing items while standing with rolling walker at sink while adhering to total hip precautions.
STG #3: By 4th session, client will safely bathe her peri area modified Ⓘ utilizing adaptive techniques and devices and 100% adherence to hip precautions.	1. Instruct in use of adaptive techniques/devices followed by demonstration of use in bathing activities. 2. Instruct in manipulation of clothing and bathing items while standing with rolling walker at sink while adhering to total hip precautions. 3. Assess for DME/home equipment needs and continued home care services if progress warrants discharge to home.

Functional Problem Statement #2: ↓ dynamic balance makes client unsafe during ADL tasks.

LTG #2: By anticipated discharge on 9/7/12, client will demonstrate safe toileting with modified Ⓘ using rolling walker and bedside commode.

Short-Term Goals	Interventions
STG #1: By next treatment session, client will transfer SBA sit ↔ stand using bedside commode and rolling walker and will manage clothing with no more than 2 verbal cues.	1. Instruct client in safe transfer techniques; reinforce compliance with total hip precautions. 2. Provide UE strengthening through reaching and weightbearing activities at sink and closet for grooming and dressing tasks and pushing up from chair and bedside commode.
STG #2: By 4th session, client will perform toileting with SBA using commode frame over toilet, grab bar, and wheeled walker, while adhering to total hip precautions.	1. Continue instruction in safe transfer techniques; reinforce compliance with total hip precautions. 2. Interview client regarding physical layout of home environment. Assess and discuss DME/adaptive equipment needs and placement in home. Explore possible interim living arrangements, family support and educate client about community support services (e.g., Meals on Wheels, elderly transit) if discharge to home is warranted.

Outpatient Rehabilitation: Cancer Intervention Plan

Name: Carol M.   **Age**: 35   **Primary Dx**: Ⓛ mastectomy 2° breast CA

Strengths: Prior to surgery, Carol was in good physical condition and employed full time as a library clerk. She has some social support from her sister who lives in another state.

Functional Problem Statement #1: Carol avoids social outings with friends due to ↓ self-esteem secondary to cosmetic alterations imposed by mastectomy procedure, which precludes her ability to return to work.

LTG #1: Carol will ↑ social interactions and activity to six outings/month within the next month, in preparation for return to work.

STGs (Objectives)	Interventions (Gateley & Borcherding, 2012)
STG #1: Carol will identify one support group of interest to her within 1 week in order to ↑ willingness to be out in public for work and social activities.	1. Educate Carol and provide written handouts re: available support groups and peer visitation groups, their contact persons and telephone numbers
STG #2: Carol will attend 1 support group activity within 2 weeks in order to ↑ confidence in social and work situations.	1. Discuss with Carol her experiences with support groups. 2. Reminder phone call or e-mail to encourage attendance at support group.
STG #3: Carol will initiate conversation with at least one other support group member during her first visit to the group in order to ↓ negative impact of cosmetic alterations to body image.	1. Accompany Carol into the community the first time she goes out. 2. Encourage Carol to participate in group discussion.
STG #4: Carol will enroll in a women's exercise program in order to ↑ activity tolerance and positive body image within 10 days.	1. Educate Carol re: area exercise groups for clients who are post-mastectomy. 2. Follow-up phone call or e-mail to determine her exercise program enrollment.
STG #5: By next session, Carol will identify five assets she possesses other than physical in order to increase self-esteem and improve confidence in social and work situations.	1. Discuss Carol's assets with her, encouraging her to think of as many as she can. 2. Educate and provide written handouts of resources (Web sites, books, organizations) that address post-mastectomy concerns.

Functional Problem Statement #2: Carol is unable to return to work 2° Ⓛ UE 3/4 AROM, 4-/5 muscle strength, ↓ activity tolerance (fatigues after 1 hr.), and sensory changes.

LTG #2: Carol will return to work part time by 3/8/13.

STGs (Objectives)	Interventions (Gateley & Borcherding, 2012)
STG #1: Carol will demonstrate activity tolerance of 2 hours for work tasks within 3 weeks.	1. Scar massage and myofascial release to incision area along with client education on self-massage. 2. Instruction in self-ranging HEP. 3. Work reconditioning tasks/job simulation
STG #2: In order to perform work task of retrieving and placing books on overhead shelves, Carol will demonstrate ↑ of 20° in Ⓛ shoulder flexion within 2 wks.	1. PROM to Ⓛ shoulder 2. Instruction in self-ranging HEP. 3. Work reconditioning tasks. 4. Provide information and encourage participation in women's exercise group.

STG #3: In order to manage repetitive work tasks, Carol will transport fifteen 5-lb boxes 10 feet (from a table to shoulder level shelf) with reported pain level of less than 2/10 within 4 wks.	1. Active resistive ROM to Ⓛ UE. 2. Resistive strengthening with exercise bands, weights, and graded functional activities. 3. Work simulation with client education on energy conservation principles. 4. Provide home exercise program and modify as client progresses. 5. Encourage participation in women's exercise group.
STG #4: Carol will use correct body mechanics in seated and active work tasks in order to have pain level of <2/10 while working within 3 wks.	1. Educate in ergonomics and posture in order to prevent pain. 2. Provide written handouts. 3. Complete work simulation tasks.
STG #5: Carol will demonstrate sensory precautions in work and daily living tasks within 10 days.	1. Provide education on safety concerns with sensory loss. 2. IADL and work-simulation tasks to assess and facilitate application of adaptive techniques for sensory hazards.

Progress Note: Hand Therapy Clinic

Date: 2/11/13   **Time**: 1:00 PM
Occupational Therapy Progress Note

S: Client reports pain at the ulnar styloid with forearm supination. Client reports she is still unable to start her car with her Ⓡ hand but can now use it to turn a doorknob.

O: Client participated in 45-minute therapy session to increase functional range of motion in Ⓡ UE for IADLs. Moist heat applied to Ⓡ hand and forearm for 10 minutes prior to beginning treatment. A/PROM Ⓡ hand and forearm were reassessed:

Ⓡ Hand	MP	PIP	DIP
Index	0/90	0/105	0/75
Long	0/90	0/105	0/80
Ring	0/90	0/105	0/80
Small	0/85	-14/105 (0/105)	0/79

[KEY: flexion/extension; ( ) PROM; - extension lag; + hyperextension]

Ⓡ Wrist: ext/flex +45/40 (+60/50)
Ⓡ forearm: supination 62 (78)   Pronation 90
Client performed the following exercises with Ⓡ UE:
Isometric forearm supination x10, AAROM supination x5, AROM forearm supination x5 followed by functional activities (carrying a tray and turning pages in a binder). Following exercises, client's supination ↑ to 77° AROM. HEP revised to include blue foam for finger flexion strengthening 2 to 3 x daily.

A: Client's gains in DIP flexion AROM since last week is due to ↑ strength of flexors. Active wrist extension ↑ 9° and flexion ↑ 5° from last week. ↑ in active pronation is due to ↑ strength while client lost 14° of forearm supination since last week, which appears to be a result of muscle tightness. Client would benefit from continued skilled OT to regain functional AROM to complete IADLs and for general strengthening.

P: Client to continue OT 2 x wk for 30-minute sessions. Continue wrist exercises and modify intervention plan to include more supination stretching and strengthening. Client will demonstrate Ⓘ in HEP and sufficient ↑ in Ⓡ forearm supination to start her car with Ⓡ UE in 2 weeks.

Laurie D., OTR/L

Contact Note: Acute Care (SOAP Format)

Date: 8/22/12   **Time**: 15:00

Occupational Therapy Contact Note

- **S:** Client nonverbal. Client demonstrated startle response with position change.
- **O:** Client participated in OT bedside 20 minutes to work on initiating and attending to self-care tasks. When asked to point finger, client required multiple verbal cues and demonstrations, and demonstrated poor response time. Client required max Ⓐ supine → sit EOB. Client also required multiple verbal cues and hand-over-hand Ⓐ 75% of the time to initiate holding on to wash cloth. Client able to bring wash cloth to water with one verbal cue but required hand-over-hand Ⓐ to bring wash cloth to face. Client attended to looking at self in mirror for ~1 minute. Client required hand-over-hand Ⓐ to initiate brushing hair. AROM shoulder flexion and abduction lack 45° at end range due to ↑ tone.
- **A:** Overall, client's motor planning, task initiation, and attention during treatment activities continues to be limited. Client would benefit from therapeutic activities to increase shoulder ROM, as well as further interventions focusing on the skills of initiating and attending to task in order to complete ADL activities.
- **P:** Client to continue OT daily for 20-minute sessions until discharge in ~4 weeks to work on self-care activities and the underlying performance skills and client factors necessary to complete tasks Ⓘ. Client will follow a one-step command in 1 week in order to attend to self-care routine.

Susan S., OTR/L

Contact Note: Acute Care (Narrative Format)

Date: 8/22/12   **Time**: 15:00

Occupational Therapy Contact Note

Client participated in OT bedside 20 minutes to work on initiating and attending to self-care tasks. Client is nonverbal and demonstrated startle response with position change. When asked to point finger, client required multiple verbal cues and demonstrations, and he demonstrated poor response time. Client required max Ⓐ supine → sit EOB. Client also required multiple verbal cues and hand-over-hand Ⓐ 75% of the time to initiate holding on to wash cloth. Client able to bring wash cloth to water with one verbal cue but required hand-over-hand Ⓐ to bring wash cloth to face. Client attended to looking at self in mirror for ~1 minute. Client required hand-over-hand Ⓐ to initiate brushing hair. AROM shoulder flexion and abduction lack 45° at end range due to ↑ tone. Overall, client's motor planning, task initiation, and attention during treatment activities continues to be limited. Client would benefit from therapeutic activities to increase shoulder ROM, as well as further interventions focusing on the skills of initiating and attending to task in order to complete ADL activities. Client to continue OT daily for 20-minute sessions until discharge in ~4 weeks to work on self-care activities and the underlying performance skills and client factors necessary to complete tasks Ⓘ. Client will follow a one-step command in 1 week in order to attend to self-care routine.

Susan S., OTR/L

Contact Note: Cognition

Date: 9/5/12   **Time**: 10:00 AM

Occupational Therapy Contact Note

- **S:** Veteran reported feeling fine, but stated he does not remember the OTA's name that he has been working with.
- **O:** In OT clinic, veteran participated in 30-minute session to improve cognition, ® UE AROM, strength, and fine motor coordination for ADLs. Veteran oriented to person, month, year, and place after two verbal cues. He followed two-step commands after max verbal cues and required mod physical assist to complete basic self-care tasks. Veteran was unable to grasp and release items with ® hand. He required mod physical Ⓐ and verbal cues to complete ® UE AROM used in tabletop activities.
- **A:** Veteran is not oriented to surroundings at all times, which presents safety concerns. His ↓ cognitive functioning leads to ↓ attention to completion of tasks, specifically dressing, feeding, and bathing. Veteran would benefit from further cognitive skills training and safety instruction. Veteran also displays ↓ strength, coordination, and AROM in ® UE, which limits his ability to complete ADL activities. He would benefit from instruction in using ® UE as an assist as well as from activities to ↑ ® UE strength, AROM, and coordination to perform self-care activities.
- **P:** Veteran to continue OT daily 1 hour for 4 weeks to improve cognitive skills, ↑ attention to task and safety awareness, and to ↑ ® UE strength, AROM, and coordination in order to complete self-care tasks. Next session, instruct client in use of calendar/daily schedule placed in room and work on improving task attention and integration of ® UE during breakfast and grooming tasks.

Duane T., COTA   Patty N., OTR/L

Contact Note: Home Health Visit

Date: 7/4/12   **Time**: 9:30 AM

Occupational Therapy Contact Note

- **S:** Client stated that he did not sleep well last night and is feeling tired this morning. Client's daughter reported that client is "transferring a little better."
- **O:** Client participated in 45-minute session in his home for skilled instruction in BADLs, safety, transfers, and use of adaptive equipment. Client and daughter were instructed in use of transfer tub bench. Following demonstration, daughter demonstrated ability to transfer client safely w/c ↔ tub bench with client needing min assist for balance and to bring legs over edge of tub. Following set-up, client was able to sequence steps for bathing but required min assist to wash back and feet using long handle sponge. Recommended that client install grab bars in tub area for safety. Client stated he will ask his nephew, who is a carpenter, to do this ASAP.
- **A:** Client demonstrates good progress in transfers from mod to min Ⓐ as compared to last week. Client's daughter demonstrates good carryover in safe transfer techniques. Client would benefit from further skilled OT instruction in transfers, self-care activities, and adaptive equipment to increase Ⓘ in home environment.
- **P:** Client to continue OT 2 x wk for 45 minutes for transfer training, activities to promote self-care Ⓘ, and family education. Client will demonstrate transfers to tub bench modified Ⓘ with use of grab bar within three treatment sessions.

Jeanine F., COTA   Leah S., OTR/L

Contact Note: Inpatient Mental Health

Date: 4/16/12   **Time**: 4:00 pm
Occupational Therapy Contact Note

S: Client reported she is currently not volunteering and has not worked for the past 4 years due to her disability status. Regarding volunteering, she says, "I need the structure," and further stated that she wants to be productive. Currently, client reports she sleeps "too much" and is having relationship problems.

O: Client was admitted yesterday and attended 4/4 group sessions today. During expressive therapy group, client participated in baking with the rest of the group, but did not eat anything. When each group member identified current emotions, client identified hers as miserable, angry, very anxious, overstimulated, frustrated, frightened, and alienated. During skills group, client identified a possible problem she may encounter upon discharge as "lack of organization," with her "red flags" being oversleeping and agitation. Client welcomed suggestions from others regarding restructuring her use of time.

A: Client is very perceptive of her emotions and limitations. Her refusal to eat with the group indicates continued appetite disturbance. Client would benefit from information about eating disorders. She would also benefit from continued group participation, with emphasis on increasing self-esteem and time management skills. Client's participation in all four group sessions today indicates good rehab potential.

P: Client will continue to attend all daily group sessions while on the acute unit to work on increasing self-esteem and ability to structure her time. Client will work on increased time management skills by developing five strategies she will use for gaining control of her daily time prior to discharge.

Nancy B., OTR/L

Contact Note: Pediatric (Preschool Age)

Date: 4/7/12   **Time**: 3 pm
Occupational Therapy Contact Note

S: Mary said she wanted to play, but when the task was difficult for her, she said, "You do it. You fix it."

O: Mary participated in 30-minute OT session in her home to work on prerequisite skills to self-care and play including: bilateral use of UEs to ↑ spontaneous use of Ⓛ hand as a functional assist, sitting balance while tailor sitting unsupported, and functional mobility. Mary was engaged during ~90% of the session.
        Bilateral UE Use: Mary required max Ⓐ to pull shirt over stuffed animal's arms with Ⓡ UE while holding it with Ⓛ UE. She spontaneously used Ⓛ hand to assist with stabilizing animal while pulling sleeve over its arm and shoulder with Ⓡ hand. Mary initiated snapping shirt, but needed max Ⓐ to use Ⓛ hand to stabilize shirt while fastening snaps. Both hands used to hold animal steady during play.
        Sitting Balance: Mary required five tactile cues from stand → sit using walker and mod physical Ⓐ from side sit → cross legged sit. She demonstrated adequate sitting balance to play for 5 minutes, requiring tactile cues twice to right herself from a lateral tilt.

A: Mary demonstrated bilateral integration and use of Ⓛ hand as a functional assist ~60% of the time, which is an increase from last week. When she is engrossed in activity, Mary is unable to concentrate on postural support and needs CGA assist to resume upright posture. She would benefit from continued skilled OT for activities that challenge postural support in order to gain protective responses, body righting, and vestibular integration in order to ↑ her Ⓘ during play.

P: Mary will continue OT weekly for 7 weeks to continue strengthening postural support in order to ↑ Ⓘ in play activities, promote bilateral hand use, and ↑ use of the Ⓛ hand as a functional assist during ADLs and play activities.

Julie S., OTR/L

Contact Note: Public School

Date: 5/12/12   **Time:** 2:30 pm
Occupational Therapy Contact Note

S: Heather did not use verbal language to communicate, but did echo words spoken to her.

O: Heather participated in 25-minute OT session in classroom to improve fine motor skills needed for scissors use and writing. After 5 minutes of brushing to decrease tactile sensitivity, Heather worked on palmar pinch and tripod grasp prehension patterns using a "Fruit Loop" bracelet activity for 20 minutes. Heather used tongs (in preparation for scissors use) to pull 15 Fruit Loops out of a cup one at a time. Then, using a palmar pinch, she placed each Fruit Loop over a pipe cleaner. 5 verbal cues were required for task completion.

A: Heather manipulates tongs well and exhibits a good awareness of positioning of tongs within her hands, which is an indicator that proper scissors use will be attained soon. Good attention to task for entire 25 minutes is an asset for completion of classroom craft projects.

P: Continue prehension activities 3 x wk using a variety of media in 20- to 30-minute intervals until proper scissors use goal is achieved. Heather will be able to cut a piece of 8-in. x 10-in. paper ~ in half using adaptive spring scissors Ⓘ 3/3 tries by the end of the school year.

Durwood T., OTR/L

Contact Note: Outpatient Clinic—Splint (SOAP Format)

Date: 9/21/12   **Time:** 1:15 pm
Occupational Therapy Contact Note

S: Client stated that the Ⓡ cock-up splint he was issued last session is not causing any problems. Client also reported that he wore splint "all day at work" for the past 3 days.

O: Client participated in 45-minute session in OT clinic for assessment of splint use/tolerance and instruction in ergonomics. Client arrived at clinic wearing splint. Skin checked following splint removal and no pressure areas noted. Client demonstrated ability to don/doff splint Ⓘ. New stockinette liner issued per client request. Client stated improvement in Ⓡ hand with a reported pain level of 3/10 (was 6/10 last week). Client was instructed in use of ergonomic equipment (split keyboard and wrist rest) for his job as a computer programmer. Following skilled instruction, client was able to demonstrate appropriate use of ergonomic devices while wearing splint. Client also provided with a catalog of ergonomic devices.

A: Client's ↓ pain from 6/10 to 3/10 since wearing splint shows good progress. Client would benefit from continued instruction in ergonomics to enable maximal performance of work tasks.

P: Continue therapy 1x weekly for 4 weeks for instruction in ergonomics, median nerve gliding exercises, and assessment of splint use/tolerance to enable work performance.

Mary J., COTA   Thomas B., OTR/L

Contact Note: Outpatient Clinic—Splint (Narrative Format)

Date: 9/21/12   **Time:** 1:15 pm
Occupational Therapy Contact Note

Client arrived at clinic wearing Ⓡ cock-up splint he was issued last session. He stated splint is not causing any problems and also reported that he wore splint "all day at work" for the past 3 days. Client then participated in 45-minute session for assessment of splint use/tolerance and instruction in ergonomics. Skin was checked following splint removal and no pressure areas noted. Client demonstrated ability to don/doff splint Ⓘ. New stockinette liner issued per client request. Client stated improvement in Ⓡ hand with a reported pain level of 3/10 (was 6/10 last week). Client was instructed in use of ergonomic equipment (split keyboard and wrist rest) for his job as a computer programmer. Following skilled instruction, client was able to demonstrate appropriate use of ergonomic devices while wearing splint. Client also provided with a catalog of ergonomic devices. Client's reduction in pain from 6/10 to 3/10 since wearing splint shows good progress. Client will benefit from continued OT 1x weekly for 4 weeks for instruction in ergonomics, median nerve gliding exercises, assessment of splint use and splint tolerance in order to enable work performance.

Mary J., COTA   Thomas B., OTR/L

Contact Note: Wheelchair Mobility Instruction (SOAP Format)

Date: 11/5/12   **Time**: 2:00 pm
Occupational Therapy Contact Note

S: Client stated, "I can't wait to try out my new power wheelchair."

O: Client participated in 75-minute session in OT clinic for instruction in use of new power w/c. Client was instructed in operating joystick control with Ⓡ hand using wrist stabilization splint. Following skilled instruction, client demonstrated ability to navigate w/c safely around obstacles, turn, and maneuver in tight spaces (i.e., bathroom). Client leaned to Ⓛ with posterior pelvic tilt when operating w/c. Preliminary instruction also provided for charging battery and care and maintenance of w/c.

A: Client demonstrates good potential for full Ⓘ in use and care of w/c. He would benefit from Ⓛ lateral w/c support, continued instruction and practice regarding charging battery, and assessment of w/c mobility on uneven surfaces.

P: Continue OT daily until discharge in 3 days for further instruction in use of power w/c. By discharge, client will demonstrate Ⓘ in w/c mobility outdoors on uneven surfaces and will maintain upright posture in w/c with use of appropriate supports.

Richard T., COTA   James F., OTR/L

Contact Note: Wheelchair Mobility Instruction (Narrative Format)

Date: 11/5/12   **Time**: 2:00 pm
Occupational Therapy Contact Note

Client stated, "I can't wait to try out my new power wheelchair" and participated in 75-minute session in OT clinic to learn how to use it. Client was instructed in operating joystick control with Ⓡ hand using wrist stabilization splint. Following skilled instruction, client demonstrated ability to navigate w/c safely around obstacles, turn, and maneuver in tight spaces (i.e., bathroom). Preliminary instruction also provided for charging battery and care and maintenance of w/c. Client leaned to Ⓛ with posterior pelvic tilt when operating w/c and would benefit from a Ⓛ lateral w/c support. Client demonstrates good potential for full Ⓘ in use and care of w/c but requires further instruction and practice regarding w/c positioning and charging battery. Continue OT daily until discharge in 3 days for further instruction in use of power w/c and assessment of w/c mobility on uneven surfaces. By discharge, client will demonstrate Ⓘ in w/c mobility outdoors on uneven surfaces and will maintain upright posture in w/c with use of appropriate supports.

Richard T., COTA   James F., OTR/L

Medicare & Medicaid Services. (2003a). *Medicare benefit policy manual* (Pub. 100-02: Ch. 7, Section altimore, MD: Author. Retrieved from http://www.cms.gov/Regulations-and-Guidance/Guidance/Downloads/bp102c07.pdf

Medicare & Medicaid Services. (2003b). *Medicare benefit policy manual* (Pub. 100-02: Ch. 7, Section Baltimore, MD: Author. Retrieved from http://www.cms.gov/Regulations-and-Guidance/Guidance/Downloads/bp102c07.pdf

Medicare & Medicaid Services. (2003c). *Medicare benefit policy manual* (Pub. 100-02: Ch. 7, Section 30.3). e, MD: Author. Retrieved from http://www.cms.gov/Regulations-and-Guidance/Guidance/Manuals/ds/bp102c07.pdf

Medicare & Medicaid Services. (2003d). *Medicare benefit policy manual* (Pub. 100-02: Ch. 7, Section Baltimore, MD: Author. Retrieved from http://www.cms.gov/Regulations-and-Guidance/Guidance/Downloads/bp102c07.pdf

Medicare & Medicaid Services. (2003e). *Medicare claims processing manual* (Pub. 100-04: Ch. 5, Section altimore, MD: Author. Retrieved from http://www.cms.gov/Regulations-and-Guidance/Guidance/downloads//clm104c05.pdf

Medicare & Medicaid Services. (2003f). *Medicare claims processing manual* (Pub. 100-04: Ch. 5, Section Baltimore, MD: Author. Retrieved from http://www.cms.gov/Regulations-and-Guidance/Guidance/downloads//clm104c05.pdf

Medicare & Medicaid Services. (2005a). *Medicare benefit policy manual* (Pub. 100-02: Ch. 15, Section Baltimore, MD: Author. Retrieved from http://www.cms.gov/Regulations-and-Guidance/Guidance/Downloads/bp102c15.pdf

Medicare & Medicaid Services. (2005b). *Medicare benefit policy manual* (Pub. 100-02: Ch. 15, Section Baltimore, MD: Author. Retrieved from http://www.cms.gov/Regulations-and-Guidance/Guidance/s/Downloads/bp102c15.pdf

Medicare & Medicaid Services. (2006a). *Medicare benefit policy manual* (Pub. 100-02: Ch. 15, Section Baltimore, MD: Author. Retrieved from http://www.cms.gov/Regulations-and-Guidance/Guidance/s/Downloads/bp102c15.pdf

r Medicare & Medicaid Services. (2006b). *Medicare benefit policy manual* (Pub. 100-02: Ch. 15, 230). Baltimore, MD: Author. Retrieved from http://www.cms.gov/Regulations-and-Guidance/Guidance/s/Downloads/bp102c15.pdf

r Medicare & Medicaid Services. (2008a). *Medicare benefit policy manual* (Pub. 100-02: Ch. 15, 220). Baltimore, MD: Author. Retrieved from http://www.cms.gov/Regulations-and-Guidance/Guidance/s/Downloads/bp102c15.pdf

r Medicare & Medicaid Services. (2008b). *Medicare benefit policy manual* (Pub. 100-02: Ch. 15, Section . Baltimore, MD: Author. Retrieved from http://www.cms.gov/Regulations-and-Guidance/Guidance/s/Downloads/bp102c15.pdf

r Medicare & Medicaid Services. (2008c). *Medicare benefit policy manual* (Pub. 100-02: Ch. 15, Section . Baltimore, MD: Author. Retrieved from http://www.cms.gov/Regulations-and-Guidance/Guidance/s/Downloads/bp102c15.pdf

r Medicare & Medicaid Services. (2008d). *Medicare benefit policy manual* (Pub. 100-02: Ch. 15, Section Baltimore, MD: Author. Retrieved from http://www.cms.gov/Regulations-and-Guidance/Guidance/ls/Downloads/bp102c15.pdf

r Medicare & Medicaid Services. (2008e). *Medicare benefit policy manual* (Pub. 100-02: Ch. 15, Section Baltimore, MD: Author. Retrieved from http://www.cms.gov/Regulations-and-Guidance/Guidance/ls/Downloads/bp102c15.pdf

r Medicare & Medicaid Services. (2009a). *11 Part B billing scenarios for PTs and OTs*. Baltimore, MD: . Retrieved from http://www.cms.gov/Medicare/Billing/TherapyServices/downloads/11_Part_B_Billing_ios_for_PTs_and_OTs.pdf

r Medicare & Medicaid Services. (2009b). *Medicare claims processing manual* (Pub. 100-04: Ch. 5, Section ltimore, MD: Author. Retrieved from http://www.cms.gov/Regulations-and-Guidance/Guidance/Manuals/oads//clm104c05.pdf

r Medicare & Medicaid Services. (2010a). *Medicare claims processing manual* (Pub. 100-04: Ch. 5, Section ltimore, MD: Author. Retrieved from http://www.cms.gov/Regulations-and-Guidance/Guidance/Manuals/oads//clm104c05.pdf

References

Accreditation Council for Occupational Therapy Education. (2012). 2011 Accredi
Therapy Education (ACOTE) Standards. *American Journal of Occupational Th*
10.5014/ajot.2012.66S6

American Academy of Professional Coders. (2012a). ICD-10 overview. Retrieved f
10/icd-10.aspx

American Academy of Professional Coders. (2012b). What is HCPCS? Retrieved from
es/medical-coding/hcpcs.aspx

American Occupational Therapy Association. (2008a). Guidelines for document
American Journal of Occupational Therapy, 62(6), 684-690.

American Occupational Therapy Association. (2008b). Occupational therapy practic
cess (2nd ed.). *American Journal of Occupational Therapy, 62*(6), 625-683.

American Occupational Therapy Association. (2008c). Occupational therapy services
the prevention of disease and disability. *American Journal of Occupational Therap*

American Occupational Therapy Association. (2009). Guidelines for supervision, ro
the delivery of occupational therapy services. *American Journal of Occupational T*

American Occupational Therapy Association. (2010a). Occupational therapy code
(2010). *American Journal of Occupational Therapy, 64*(6 Suppl.), S17-S26. doi: 10.5

American Occupational Therapy Association. (2010b). Scope of practice. *American Jo*
64(Suppl.), S70-S77. doi: 10.5014/ajot.2010.64S70

American Occupational Therapy Association. (2010c). Standards of practice for oc
Journal of Occupational Therapy, 64(6 Suppl.), S106-S111. doi: 10.5014/ajot.2010.64

American Occupational Therapy Association. (2011). Fact sheet: Occupational the
recovery. Retrieved from http://www.aota.org/Consumers/Professionals/WhatIs
aspx?FT=.pdf

American Occupational Therapy Association. (2012). Physical agent modalities. *Ame*
Therapy, 66(6 Suppl.), S78-S80. doi: 10.5014/ajot.2012.66S78

American Psychological Association. (2010). *Publication manual of the American Psyc*
Washington, DC: Author.

Centers for
30.1.1).
Manuals
Centers for
30.1.2).
Manual
Centers for
Baltimo
Downlo
Centers for
40.2.4.3
Manual
Centers for
20.3). I
Manual
Centers fo
100.2).
Manual
Centers fo
220.1).
Manual
Centers fo
220.1.1)
Manua
Centers fc
220.2).
Manua
Centers f
Section
Manua
Centers f
Section
Manua
Centers fe
220.1.2
Manu
Centers f
220.1.
Manu
Centers f
220.3)
Manu
Centers
230.2)
Manu
Centers
Autho
Scena
Centers
20). B
down
Centers
10). B
down

References

Accreditation Council for Occupational Therapy Education. (2012). 2011 Accreditation Council for Occupational Therapy Education (ACOTE) Standards. *American Journal of Occupational Therapy, 66*(6 Suppl.), S6-S74. doi: 10.5014/ajot.2012.66S6

American Academy of Professional Coders. (2012a). ICD-10 overview. Retrieved from http://www.aapc.com/ICD-10/icd-10.aspx

American Academy of Professional Coders. (2012b). What is HCPCS? Retrieved from http://www.aapc.com/resources/medical-coding/hcpcs.aspx

American Occupational Therapy Association. (2008a). Guidelines for documentation of occupational therapy. *American Journal of Occupational Therapy, 62*(6), 684-690.

American Occupational Therapy Association. (2008b). Occupational therapy practice framework: Domain and process (2nd ed.). *American Journal of Occupational Therapy, 62*(6), 625-683.

American Occupational Therapy Association. (2008c). Occupational therapy services in the promotion of health and the prevention of disease and disability. *American Journal of Occupational Therapy, 62*(6), 694-703.

American Occupational Therapy Association. (2009). Guidelines for supervision, roles, and responsibilities during the delivery of occupational therapy services. *American Journal of Occupational Therapy, 63*(6), 797-803.

American Occupational Therapy Association. (2010a). Occupational therapy code of ethics and ethics standards (2010). *American Journal of Occupational Therapy, 64*(6 Suppl.), S17-S26. doi: 10.5014/ajot.2010.64S17

American Occupational Therapy Association. (2010b). Scope of practice. *American Journal of Occupational Therapy, 64*(Suppl.), S70-S77. doi: 10.5014/ajot.2010.64S70

American Occupational Therapy Association. (2010c). Standards of practice for occupational therapy. *American Journal of Occupational Therapy, 64*(6 Suppl.), S106-S111. doi: 10.5014/ajot.2010.64S106

American Occupational Therapy Association. (2011). Fact sheet: Occupational therapy's role in mental health recovery. Retrieved from http://www.aota.org/Consumers/Professionals/WhatIsOT/MH/Facts/MH-Recovery.aspx?FT=.pdf

American Occupational Therapy Association. (2012). Physical agent modalities. *American Journal of Occupational Therapy, 66*(6 Suppl.), S78-S80. doi: 10.5014/ajot.2012.66S78

American Psychological Association. (2010). *Publication manual of the American Psychological Association* (6th ed.). Washington, DC: Author.

Morreale MJ, Borcherding S.
The OTA's Guide to Documentation:
Writing SOAP Notes, Third Edition (pp 191-194).
© 2013 SLACK Incorporated.

Centers for Medicare & Medicaid Services. (2003a). *Medicare benefit policy manual* (Pub. 100-02: Ch. 7, Section 30.1.1). Baltimore, MD: Author. Retrieved from http://www.cms.gov/Regulations-and-Guidance/Guidance/Manuals/Downloads/bp102c07.pdf

Centers for Medicare & Medicaid Services. (2003b). *Medicare benefit policy manual* (Pub. 100-02: Ch. 7, Section 30.1.2). Baltimore, MD: Author. Retrieved from http://www.cms.gov/Regulations-and-Guidance/Guidance/Manuals/Downloads/bp102c07.pdf

Centers for Medicare & Medicaid Services. (2003c). *Medicare benefit policy manual* (Pub. 100-02: Ch. 7, Section 30.3). Baltimore, MD: Author. Retrieved from http://www.cms.gov/Regulations-and-Guidance/Guidance/Manuals/Downloads/bp102c07.pdf

Centers for Medicare & Medicaid Services. (2003d). *Medicare benefit policy manual* (Pub. 100-02: Ch. 7, Section 40.2.4.3. Baltimore, MD: Author. Retrieved from http://www.cms.gov/Regulations-and-Guidance/Guidance/Manuals/Downloads/bp102c07.pdf

Centers for Medicare & Medicaid Services. (2003e). *Medicare claims processing manual* (Pub. 100-04: Ch. 5, Section 20.3). Baltimore, MD: Author. Retrieved from http://www.cms.gov/Regulations-and-Guidance/Guidance/Manuals/downloads//clm104c05.pdf

Centers for Medicare & Medicaid Services. (2003f). *Medicare claims processing manual* (Pub. 100-04: Ch. 5, Section 100.2). Baltimore, MD: Author. Retrieved from http://www.cms.gov/Regulations-and-Guidance/Guidance/Manuals/downloads//clm104c05.pdf

Centers for Medicare & Medicaid Services. (2005a). *Medicare benefit policy manual* (Pub. 100-02: Ch. 15, Section 220.1). Baltimore, MD: Author. Retrieved from http://www.cms.gov/Regulations-and-Guidance/Guidance/Manuals/Downloads/bp102c15.pdf

Centers for Medicare & Medicaid Services. (2005b). *Medicare benefit policy manual* (Pub. 100-02: Ch. 15, Section 220.1.1). Baltimore, MD: Author. Retrieved from http://www.cms.gov/Regulations-and-Guidance/Guidance/Manuals/Downloads/bp102c15.pdf

Centers for Medicare & Medicaid Services. (2006a). *Medicare benefit policy manual* (Pub. 100-02: Ch. 15, Section 220.2). Baltimore, MD: Author. Retrieved from http://www.cms.gov/Regulations-and-Guidance/Guidance/Manuals/Downloads/bp102c15.pdf

Centers for Medicare & Medicaid Services. (2006b). *Medicare benefit policy manual* (Pub. 100-02: Ch. 15, Section 230). Baltimore, MD: Author. Retrieved from http://www.cms.gov/Regulations-and-Guidance/Guidance/Manuals/Downloads/bp102c15.pdf

Centers for Medicare & Medicaid Services. (2008a). *Medicare benefit policy manual* (Pub. 100-02: Ch. 15, Section 220). Baltimore, MD: Author. Retrieved from http://www.cms.gov/Regulations-and-Guidance/Guidance/Manuals/Downloads/bp102c15.pdf

Centers for Medicare & Medicaid Services. (2008b). *Medicare benefit policy manual* (Pub. 100-02: Ch. 15, Section 220.1.2). Baltimore, MD: Author. Retrieved from http://www.cms.gov/Regulations-and-Guidance/Guidance/Manuals/Downloads/bp102c15.pdf

Centers for Medicare & Medicaid Services. (2008c). *Medicare benefit policy manual* (Pub. 100-02: Ch. 15, Section 220.1.3). Baltimore, MD: Author. Retrieved from http://www.cms.gov/Regulations-and-Guidance/Guidance/Manuals/Downloads/bp102c15.pdf

Centers for Medicare & Medicaid Services. (2008d). *Medicare benefit policy manual* (Pub. 100-02: Ch. 15, Section 220.3). Baltimore, MD: Author. Retrieved from http://www.cms.gov/Regulations-and-Guidance/Guidance/Manuals/Downloads/bp102c15.pdf

Centers for Medicare & Medicaid Services. (2008e). *Medicare benefit policy manual* (Pub. 100-02: Ch. 15, Section 230.2). Baltimore, MD: Author. Retrieved from http://www.cms.gov/Regulations-and-Guidance/Guidance/Manuals/Downloads/bp102c15.pdf

Centers for Medicare & Medicaid Services. (2009a). *11 Part B billing scenarios for PTs and OTs.* Baltimore, MD: Author. Retrieved from http://www.cms.gov/Medicare/Billing/TherapyServices/downloads/11_Part_B_Billing_Scenarios_for_PTs_and_OTs.pdf

Centers for Medicare & Medicaid Services. (2009b). *Medicare claims processing manual* (Pub. 100-04: Ch. 5, Section 20). Baltimore, MD: Author. Retrieved from http://www.cms.gov/Regulations-and-Guidance/Guidance/Manuals/downloads//clm104c05.pdf

Centers for Medicare & Medicaid Services. (2010a). *Medicare claims processing manual* (Pub. 100-04: Ch. 5, Section 10). Baltimore, MD: Author. Retrieved from http://www.cms.gov/Regulations-and-Guidance/Guidance/Manuals/downloads//clm104c05.pdf

Centers for Medicare & Medicaid Services. (2010b). *Medicare claims processing manual* (Pub. 100-04: Ch. 5, Section 10.2). Baltimore, MD: Author. Retrieved from http://www.cms.gov/Regulations-and-Guidance/Guidance/Manuals/downloads//clm104c05.pdf

Centers for Medicare & Medicaid Services. (2010c). *Medicare claims processing manual* (Pub. 100-04: Ch. 5, Section 10.3). Baltimore, MD: Author. Retrieved from http://www.cms.gov/Regulations-and-Guidance/Guidance/Manuals/downloads//clm104c05.pdf

Centers for Medicare & Medicaid Services. (2011a). *Medicare benefit policy manual* (Pub. 100-02: Ch. 7, Section 40.2.1). Baltimore, MD: Author. Retrieved from http://www.cms.gov/Regulations-and-Guidance/Guidance/Manuals/Downloads/bp102c07.pdf

Centers for Medicare & Medicaid Services. (2011b). *Medicare claims processing manual* (Pub. 100-04: Ch. 5, Section 20.2). Baltimore, MD: Author. Retrieved from http://www.cms.gov/Regulations-and-Guidance/Guidance/Manuals/downloads//clm104c05.pdf

Centers for Medicare & Medicaid Services. (2011c). *2012 OASIS-C guidance manual* (Chapter 1). Baltimore, MD: Author. Retrieved from http://www.cms.gov/Medicare/Quality-Initiatives-Patient-Assessment-Instruments/HomeHealthQualityInits/HHQIOASISUserManual.html

Centers for Medicare & Medicaid Services. (2012a). Accreditation. Retrieved from https://www.cms.gov/Medicare/Provider-Enrollment-and-Certification/SurveyCertificationGenInfo/Accreditation.html

Centers for Medicare & Medicaid Services. (2012b). EHR incentive programs. Retrieved from https://www.cms.gov/Regulations-and-Guidance/Legislation/EHRIncentivePrograms/index.html

Centers for Medicare & Medicaid Services. (2012c). *Long-Term Care Facility Resident Assessment Instrument User's Manual MDS 3.0 April 2012* (Ch. 1, Section 1.1). Baltimore, MD: Author. Retrieved from http://www.cms.gov/Medicare/Quality-Initiatives-Patient-Assessment-Instruments/NursingHomeQualityInits/NHQIMDS30-ArchivedRAIManuals.html

Centers for Medicare & Medicaid Services. (2012d). *Long-Term Care Facility Resident Assessment Instrument User's Manual MDS 3.0 April 2012* (Ch. 1, Section 1.2). Baltimore, MD: Author. Retrieved from http://www.cms.gov/Medicare/Quality-Initiatives-Patient-Assessment-Instruments/NursingHomeQualityInits/NHQIMDS30-ArchivedRAIManuals.html

Centers for Medicare & Medicaid Services. (2012e). *Long-Term Care Facility Resident Assessment Instrument User's Manual MDS 3.0 April 2012* (Ch. 1, Section 1.3). Baltimore, MD: Author. Retrieved from http://www.cms.gov/Medicare/Quality-Initiatives-Patient-Assessment-Instruments/NursingHomeQualityInits/NHQIMDS30-ArchivedRAIManuals.html

Centers for Medicare & Medicaid Services. (2012f). *Medicare Learning Network: Mental health services.* Baltimore, MD: Author. Retrieved from http://www.cms.gov/Outreach-and-Education/Medicare-Learning-Network-MLN/MLNProducts/downloads/Mental_Health_Services_ICN903195.pdf

Centers for Medicare & Medicaid Services. (2012g). Personal health records. Retrieved from https://www.cms.gov/Medicare/E-Health/PerHealthRecords/index.html?redirect=/PerHealthRecords/

Centers for Medicare & Medicaid Services. (2012h). *2011 actuarial report on the financial outlook for Medicaid.* Baltimore, MD: Author. Retrieved from https://www.cms.gov/Research-Statistics-Data-and-Systems/Research/ActuarialStudies/downloads/MedicaidReport2011.pdf

Centers for Medicare & Medicaid Services. (n.d.). What is Medicare? Retrieved from Medicare.gov website: http://www.medicare.gov/sign-up-change-plans/decide-how-to-get-medicare/whats-medicare/what-is-medicare.html

Clark, G. F. (2005). Developing appropriate student IEP goals. *OT Practice, 10*(14), 12-15.

Coffman-Kadish, N. (2003). Numbering and filing systems. In M. A. Skurka (Ed.), *Health information management: Principles and organization for health information services* (5th ed., pp. 105-127). San Francisco, CA: Jossey-Bass.

Fearon, H. M., Levine, S. M., & Quinn, L. (2010). Payment policy and coding. In L. Quinn & J. Gordon. *Documentation for rehabilitation: A guide to clinical decision making* (2nd ed., pp. 177-190). Maryland Heights, MO: Saunders.

Fremgen, B. F. (2009). *Medical law and ethics* (3rd ed.). Upper Saddle River, NJ: Pearson Education, Inc.

Gateley, C. A., & Borcherding, S. (2012). *Documentation manual for occupational therapy: Writing SOAP notes* (3rd ed.). Thorofare, NJ: SLACK Incorporated.

Herbold, J. (2010). Computerized documentation. In L. Quinn & J. Gordon. *Documentation for rehabilitation: A guide to clinical decision making* (2nd ed., pp. 191-201). Maryland Heights, MO: Saunders.

Institute for Safe Medication Practices. (2011). *ISMP's list of error-prone abbreviations, symbols, and dose designations.* Horsham, PA: Author. Retrieved from http://www.ismp.org/Tools/errorproneabbreviations.pdf

Joint Commission. (2012). *Facts about the official "do not use" list of abbreviations.* Oakbrook Terrace, IL: Author. Retrieved from http://www.jointcommission.org/assets/1/18/Do_Not_Use_List.pdf

Kannenberg, K., & Greene, S. (2003). Infusing occupation into practice: Valuing and supporting the psychosocial foundation of occupation. *OT Practice, 8*(10), CE-1-CE-8.

Kettenbach, G. (2009). *Writing patient/client notes: Ensuring accuracy in documentation* (4th ed.). Philadelphia, PA: F.A. Davis.

Küpper, L. (Ed.). (2012). The basics of early intervention: 9 key definitions in early intervention (Section 3 of Module 1). Building the legacy for our youngest children with disabilities: A training curriculum on Part C of IDEA 2004. Washington, DC: National Dissemination Center for Children with Disabilities. Retrieved from http://nichcy.org/laws/idea/legacy/partc/module1

Merriam-Webster. (2001). *Merriam-Webster's guide to punctuation and style* (2nd ed.). Springfield, MA: Author.

Pierson, F. M., & Fairchild, S. L. (2008). *Principles & techniques of patient care* (4th ed.). St. Louis, MO: Saunders.

Quinn, L., & Gordon, J. (2010). *Documentation for rehabilitation: A guide to clinical decision making* (2nd ed.). Maryland Heights, MO: Saunders.

Sames, K. M. (2010). *Documenting occupational therapy practice* (2nd ed.). Upper Saddle River, NJ: Pearson.

Scott, R. W. (2013). *Legal, ethical, and practical aspects of patient care documentation* (4th ed.). Burlington, MA: Jones & Bartlett Learning.

U.S. Department of Education. (2006). Topic: Individualized Education Program (IEP). Retrieved from http://idea.ed.gov/explore/view/p/%2Croot%2Cdynamic%2CTopicalBrief%2C10%2C

U.S. Department of Education. (2011). General: Family Educational Rights and Privacy Act (FERPA). Retrieved from http://www2.ed.gov/policy/gen/guid/fpco/ferpa/index.html

U.S. Department of Education. (n.d.). Model forms. Retrieved from http://idea.ed.gov/static/modelForms

U.S. Department of Health & Human Services. (2002). Incidental uses and disclosures. Retrieved from http://www.hhs.gov/ocr/privacy/hipaa/understanding/coveredentities/incidentalusesanddisclosures.html

U.S. Department of Health & Human Services. (2003a). *OCR privacy brief: Summary of the HIPAA Privacy Rule.* Washington, D.C.: Author. Retrieved from http://www.hhs.gov/ocr/privacy/hipaa/understanding/summary/privacysummary.pdf

U.S. Department of Health & Human Services. (2003b). Uses and disclosures for treatment, payment, and health care operations. Retrieved from http://www.hhs.gov/ocr/privacy/hipaa/understanding/coveredentities/usesanddisclosuresfortpo.html

U.S. Department of Health & Human Services. (2009). What do the HIPAA Privacy and Security Rules require of covered entities when they dispose of protected health information? Retrieved from http://www.hhs.gov/ocr/privacy/hipaa/faq/safeguards/575.html

World Health Organization. (2002). *Towards a common language for functioning, disability and health: ICF.* Geneva, Switzerland: Author. Retrieved from http://www.who.int/classifications/icf/training/icfbeginnersguide.pdf

World Health Organization. (2012a). Classifications: International Classification of Diseases (ICD) information sheet. Retrieved from http://www.who.int/classifications/icd/factsheet/en/index.html

World Health Organization. (2012b). Classifications: International Classification of Functioning, Disability and Health (ICF). Retrieved from http://www.who.int/classifications/icf/en/

Youngstrom, M. J. (2002). The occupational therapy practice framework: The evolution of our professional language. *American Journal of Occupational Therapy, 56*(6), 607-608.

Appendix

Suggestions for Completing the Worksheets

If you are a student, new OTA, or instructor using this manual, you should be able to work your way through the exercises and check your work against those in this Appendix. The suggestions offered here are only a few of the many possible "good" or "correct" answers. As you do the exercises, remember that your answer can be different and still be correct, as long as it contains the essential elements. You should not sacrifice your own writing style to be more like someone else's, provided your information and protocol are essentially correct. SOAP notes are difficult to write without a real treatment session. Although there are many examples in this manual, there is no substitute for observing or working with actual clients. Only then will you be able to translate your treatment session onto paper or an electronic format in a meaningful way.

Chapter 1

Worksheet 1-1: Using the *Occupational Therapy Practice Framework*

Performance skills related to a clay or craft project might include observable behaviors such as the following: activity tolerance, sharing of materials, ability to organize time and materials, sequencing of steps, task initiation, decision making, asking for assistance, reaching for objects, sitting upright, speaking with others, gathering and searching for materials, attention to detail, coordination of both hands, crossing midline, frustration tolerance, pacing of activity, following directions or pattern, handling of tools, and many others.

Client factors related to a clay or craft project might include the following: UE AROM, strength, vision, hearing, touch, attention, eye-hand coordination, spatial awareness, concept formation, self-esteem, motor planning, gait patterns, muscle tone, stamina, temperament, attitude and values regarding crafts, standards for completion, and many others.

Worksheet 1-2: *Occupational Therapy Practice Framework*—More Practice

Performance skills related to a cooking task might include behaviors such as the following: knowledge of tools and equipment; carrying objects; adapting to environment; activity tolerance; ability to organize time, materials, and steps; task initiation; clean up; judgment, safety, and problem solving; reaching for objects; mobility; dynamic balance; lifting, stabilizing, pouring, and handling objects; gathering and searching for materials; coordination of both hands; pacing of activity; following directions; and many others.

Morreale MJ, Borcherding S.
The OTA's Guide to Documentation:
Writing SOAP Notes, Third Edition (pp 195-218).
© 2013 SLACK Incorporated.

Worksheet 4-3: Deciphering Doctors' Orders and Abbreviations

1. Dx s/p Ⓡ TKR 2° OA, WBAT
   OT 2x/wk for BADLs, IADLs

   Diagnosis: status post right total knee replacement secondary to osteoarthritis, weightbearing as tolerated.

   Occupational therapy ordered two times weekly for basic and instrumental activities of daily living.

2. X-ray + Ⓛ index finger MCP Fx 2° GSW

   X-ray is positive for a left index finger metacarpophalangeal joint fracture, which is secondary to a gunshot wound.

3. 5 y.o. child has pain 2° bone CA Ⓛ LE

   Five-year-old child has pain secondary to bone cancer in left lower extremity.

4. Dx Ⓡ DRUJ Fx c̄ ORIF
   OT 3x/wk for PAMs PRN, P/AROM, ADLs, CPM

   Diagnosis is right distal radioulnar joint fracture with open reduction and internal fixation.

   Occupational therapy ordered three times weekly for physical agent modalities as needed, passive and active range of motion, activities of daily living, continuous passive motion.

5. 1° Dx PTSD, 2° Dx OCD

   Primary diagnosis is post-traumatic stress disorder; secondary diagnosis is obsessive compulsive disorder.

6. 1° Dx DJD Ⓡ hip, 2° Dx COPD & CHF

   Primary diagnosis is degenerative joint disease right hip and secondary diagnoses are chronic obstructive pulmonary disease and congestive heart failure.

7. Dx CAD, TIA

   Diagnosis is coronary artery disease and transient ischemic attack.

Worksheet 4-4: Deciphering Doctors' Orders and Abbreviations—More Practice

1. Dx PDD-NOS, ADHD
   OT: ADLs, SI, FM
   2 x/wk X 12 wks

   Diagnoses are pervasive developmental disorder not otherwise specified and attention deficit hyperactivity disorder.

   Occupational therapy ordered for activities of daily living, sensory integration, fine-motor skills.

   Twice weekly for twelve weeks.

2. EMG – Ⓡ CTS and – TOS

   Electromyogram is negative for right carpal tunnel syndrome and negative for thoracic outlet syndrome.

3. Dx: s/p Ⓛ THR, pt. NWB Ⓛ LE, OOB c̄ walker
   OT eval. and tx; ADLs, Ⓑ UE PREs
   3x/wk X 4 wks

   Diagnosis is status post left total hip replacement. Patient has non-weightbearing status for left lower extremity and may get out of bed with use of walker.

   Occupational therapy ordered for evaluation and treatment, activities of daily living, bilateral upper extremity progressive resistive exercises.

   Three times weekly for 4 weeks.

4. MRI + TBI, VS stable, BRP

   Magnetic resonance imaging is positive for traumatic brain injury. Vital signs are stable. Patient is allowed bathroom privileges (able to get out of bed and use the bathroom).

Appendix

Suggestions for Completing the Worksheets

If you are a student, new OTA, or instructor using this manual, you should be able to work your way through the exercises and check your work against those in this Appendix. The suggestions offered here are only a few of the many possible "good" or "correct" answers. As you do the exercises, remember that your answer can be different and still be correct, as long as it contains the essential elements. You should not sacrifice your own writing style to be more like someone else's, provided your information and protocol are essentially correct. SOAP notes are difficult to write without a real treatment session. Although there are many examples in this manual, there is no substitute for observing or working with actual clients. Only then will you be able to translate your treatment session onto paper or an electronic format in a meaningful way.

Chapter 1

Worksheet 1-1: Using the *Occupational Therapy Practice Framework*

Performance skills related to a clay or craft project might include observable behaviors such as the following: activity tolerance, sharing of materials, ability to organize time and materials, sequencing of steps, task initiation, decision making, asking for assistance, reaching for objects, sitting upright, speaking with others, gathering and searching for materials, attention to detail, coordination of both hands, crossing midline, frustration tolerance, pacing of activity, following directions or pattern, handling of tools, and many others.

Client factors related to a clay or craft project might include the following: UE AROM, strength, vision, hearing, touch, attention, eye-hand coordination, spatial awareness, concept formation, self-esteem, motor planning, gait patterns, muscle tone, stamina, temperament, attitude and values regarding crafts, standards for completion, and many others.

Worksheet 1-2: *Occupational Therapy Practice Framework*—More Practice

Performance skills related to a cooking task might include behaviors such as the following: knowledge of tools and equipment; carrying objects; adapting to environment; activity tolerance; ability to organize time, materials, and steps; task initiation; clean up; judgment, safety, and problem solving; reaching for objects; mobility; dynamic balance; lifting, stabilizing, pouring, and handling objects; gathering and searching for materials; coordination of both hands; pacing of activity; following directions; and many others.

Morreale MJ, Borcherding S.
The OTA's Guide to Documentation:
Writing SOAP Notes, Third Edition (pp 195-218).
© 2013 SLACK Incorporated.

Client factors related to a cooking task might include the following: appetite, attitude and values regarding food, body image, UE AROM, strength, vision, hearing, smell, touch, eye-hand coordination, spatial awareness, depth and distance perception, concept formation, learned behaviors, motor planning, gait patterns, muscle tone, stamina, temperament, standards for completion, and many others.

Worksheet 3-1: Use of Aides

1. Y Help maintain inventory of adaptive equipment and supplies.
2. Y Place completed OT paperwork in medical charts.
3. N Instruct the client in new therapy putty exercises.
4. N Instruct the client in a sliding board transfer.
5. Y Assist the OT practitioner with a client transfer.
6. N Upgrade a client's exercise program.
7. Y Photocopy a home exercise program for client's chart.
8. Y Transport a stable client in a wheelchair from his hospital room to the OT room.
9. Y While the OTA is leading a sensory group, assist a client in that group to handle tactile objects.
10. Y Assist client in filling out client information forms.
11. N Teach a client how to use lower extremity adaptive equipment following a total hip replacement.
12. N Determine what adaptive feeding equipment is needed for a client who has a CVA with right hemiparesis.
13. Y Schedule OT appointments.
14. N Select activities for a client's fine motor exercises.
15. Y Assist the OTA with client wound care by opening bandage packages and instruments.
16. N Adjust settings on a TENS unit when client reports not feeling the treatment modality work.
17. Y Sit and talk with a client while client is receiving a hot pack or other modality.
18. Y Assist a child with scissors skills when more practice is needed after child learns the task and condition is stable.
19. Y Obtain therapeutic equipment for the OTA to use with client.
20. Y Cut out Velcro tabs and straps for splint that OTA is fabricating.
21. N Administer part of a standardized assessment.
22. Y Add more paraffin to unit when paraffin levels are low.
23. Y Maintain temperature log of hydrocollator.
24. N Determine if a client should have a paraffin treatment rather than a hot pack that day.
25. Y Set up client's meal tray in preparation for OT feeding session.
26. Y Clean equipment and treatment tables/mats.
27. Y Place reality orientation calendar in client's room.
28. N Determine if a client is adhering to weight bearing precautions during morning ADLs.

Chapter 4

Worksheet 4-1: Using Abbreviations

1. Pt. Ⓘ BADLs.
   Patient is independent in basic activities of daily living.
2. Client reports ↓ pain Ⓡ shoulder p̄ HP.
   Client reports decreased pain in right shoulder following a hot pack.

3. Resident w/c ↔ EOB with SBA.

   Resident transferred from the wheelchair to edge of bed and transferred back to wheelchair with stand-by assist.

4. Client c/o pain in Ⓡ index MCP joint p̄ ~5 min PROM.

   Client complained of pain in the right index finger metacarpophalangeal joint after approximately 5 minutes of passive range of motion.

5. Client w/c → mat c̄ sliding board max Ⓐ x2.

   Client transferred from his wheelchair to the mat using a sliding board and maximum assistance of two people.

6. Pt. O x 4.

   Patient is oriented to person, place, time, and situation.

7. Client has SOB c̄ PRE.

   Client has shortness of breath when performing progressive resistive exercises.

8. Pt. has ↓ STM and OCD which limit IADLs.

   Patient has decreased short-term memory and obsessive compulsive disorder, which limit instrumental activities of daily living.

9. Pt. min Ⓐ AMB bed → toilet 2° ↓ balance.

   Patient requires minimal assistance to ambulate from bed to toilet secondary to decreased balance.

10. Child's FM WFL to don AFO.

    The child's fine motor skills are within functional limits to put on ankle-foot orthosis.

Worksheet 4-2: Using Abbreviations—Additional Practice

1. Client requires minimal assistance to stand and pull up clothing with partial weightbearing status of right lower extremity.

   Client min Ⓐ to stand and pull up clothing c̄ PWB Ⓡ LE.

2. Patient is able to feed herself independently with the use of built-up utensils.

   Pt. Ⓘ feeding c̄ built-up utensils.

3. Client has intact sensation in both upper extremities but complains of minimal pain.

   Client has intact sensation Ⓑ UE but c/o min pain.

4. Client has 55 degrees of passive range of motion in the left index distal interphalangeal joint, which is within functional limits.

   55° PROM in Ⓛ index DIP is WFL.

5. While sitting on edge of bed, client is able to put on her socks with stand-by assistance but requires moderate assistance with putting on and taking off left shoe.

   Client dons socks c̄ SBA while sitting EOB but requires mod Ⓐ to don & doff Ⓛ shoe.

6. Student is independent in wheelchair mobility and basic activities of daily living.

   Student Ⓘ w/c mobility and BADLs.

7. Patient requires moderate assistance of two people to transfer from wheelchair to toilet and from toilet to wheelchair.

   Pt. mod Ⓐ x2 w/c ↔ toilet.

8. Patient's toe-touch weightbearing status limits her performance of instrumental activities of daily living.

   Pt.'s TTWB limits IADLs.

Worksheet 4-3: Deciphering Doctors' Orders and Abbreviations

1. Dx s/p Ⓡ TKR 2° OA, WBAT
    OT 2x/wk for BADLs, IADLs

    Diagnosis: status post right total knee replacement secondary to osteoarthritis, weightbearing as tolerated.

    Occupational therapy ordered two times weekly for basic and instrumental activities of daily living.

2. X-ray + Ⓛ index finger MCP Fx 2° GSW

    X-ray is positive for a left index finger metacarpophalangeal joint fracture, which is secondary to a gunshot wound.

3. 5 y.o. child has pain 2° bone CA Ⓛ LE

    Five-year-old child has pain secondary to bone cancer in left lower extremity.

4. Dx Ⓡ DRUJ Fx c̄ ORIF
    OT 3x/wk for PAMs PRN, P/AROM, ADLs, CPM

    Diagnosis is right distal radioulnar joint fracture with open reduction and internal fixation.

    Occupational therapy ordered three times weekly for physical agent modalities as needed, passive and active range of motion, activities of daily living, continuous passive motion.

5. 1° Dx PTSD, 2° Dx OCD

    Primary diagnosis is post-traumatic stress disorder; secondary diagnosis is obsessive compulsive disorder.

6. 1° Dx DJD Ⓡ hip, 2° Dx COPD & CHF

    Primary diagnosis is degenerative joint disease right hip and secondary diagnoses are chronic obstructive pulmonary disease and congestive heart failure.

7. Dx CAD, TIA

    Diagnosis is coronary artery disease and transient ischemic attack.

Worksheet 4-4: Deciphering Doctors' Orders and Abbreviations—More Practice

1. Dx PDD-NOS, ADHD
    OT: ADLs, SI, FM
    2 x/wk X 12 wks

    Diagnoses are pervasive developmental disorder not otherwise specified and attention deficit hyperactivity disorder.

    Occupational therapy ordered for activities of daily living, sensory integration, fine-motor skills.

    Twice weekly for twelve weeks.

2. EMG – Ⓡ CTS and – TOS

    Electromyogram is negative for right carpal tunnel syndrome and negative for thoracic outlet syndrome.

3. Dx: s/p Ⓛ THR, pt. NWB Ⓛ LE, OOB c̄ walker
    OT eval. and tx; ADLs, Ⓑ UE PREs
    3x/wk X 4 wks

    Diagnosis is status post left total hip replacement. Patient has non-weightbearing status for left lower extremity and may get out of bed with use of walker.

    Occupational therapy ordered for evaluation and treatment, activities of daily living, bilateral upper extremity progressive resistive exercises.

    Three times weekly for 4 weeks.

4. MRI + TBI, VS stable, BRP

    Magnetic resonance imaging is positive for traumatic brain injury. Vital signs are stable. Patient is allowed bathroom privileges (able to get out of bed and use the bathroom).

5. CXR – TB but + URI, pt. has DOE and FUO

   Chest x-ray is negative for tuberculosis but positive for an upper respiratory infection. Patient has dyspnea upon exertion and fever of unknown origin.

6. Dx PTSD, MS, HBV

   Client's diagnoses are post-traumatic stress disorder, multiple sclerosis, and hepatitis B virus.

Worksheet 4-5: Additional Practice

1. *Pt. participated in OT session bedside for instruction in BADLs. Max Ⓐ to don LE garments, mod Ⓐ to don UE garments. Mod Ⓐ for bed mobility. Supine → sit min Ⓐ and sit → stand mod Ⓐ.*

2. *Resident to OT via w/c escort. Resident leans Ⓛ and needs verbal cues and min physical assist to maintain symmetrical posture in midline. Standing pivot transfer w/c → toilet mod Ⓐ for balance. Verbal cues and feedback using a mirror needed to maintain upright posture.*
   -or-

   Resident to OT via w/c escort. Resident leans Ⓛ and needs verbal cues and visual feedback from mirror to maintain upright symmetrical posture in midline. Standing pivot w/c → toilet mod Ⓐ for balance.

3. *Pt. 10 wks s/p Ⓛ DRUJ Fx and has an URI. Pt. participated in 40-minute session in OT clinic for assessment of relevant client factors. Strength Ⓛ shoulder and elbow flex./ext. are 4/5, wrist flex./ext. 3-/5, grip strength 8#. Light touch intact. Ⓡ UE strength and sensation WFL.*

Worksheet 4-6: Generating Abbreviations

Here are some suggestions from the abbreviations list in the book:

Lower extremity weightbearing status:
   NWB, TTWB, PWB, WBAT, FWB

Different types of range of motion:
   ROM, PROM, AROM, AAROM, TAM, TPM

Physical agent modalities:
   US, W/cm², M/Hz, HP, CPM, TENS, NMES, °C, °F, HVPC

Chapter 5

Worksheet 5-1: Quoting and Paraphrasing

1. *C*   The child stated that she was extremely hungry.
2. *I*   The child stated that "she was starving."
3. *I*   The child "stated I am starving."
4. *C*   The child indicated that she was "starving."
5. *I*   The child stated "I am starving".
6. *I*   The patient asked how to put her splint on?
7. *I*   The patient asked "How do I put my splint on"?
8. *C*   The patient asked about the proper way to put on her splint.
9. *C*   The patient asked, "How do I put my splint on?"
10. *I*   The patient asked "how to put her splint on."
11. *C*   The client requested a new buttonhook.
12. *I*   The client asked if "she could have a new buttonhook."
13. *I*   The client asked, "Can I have a new buttonhook"?

14. *C*   The client asked for a new buttonhook.
15. *C*   The client asked, "Can I have a new buttonhook?"
16. *I*   The client stated "he felt dizzy" as he stood at the kitchen counter.
17. *C*   The client reported feeling "dizzy" while standing at the kitchen counter.
18. *I*   While standing at the kitchen counter, the client stated "he felt dizzy."
19. *I*   The client, while standing at the kitchen counter, stated I feel "dizzy."
20. *C*   The client reported dizziness while standing at the kitchen counter.

Mini Worksheet 5-2: Spelling

1. ___ defered   ✓ deferred   7. ___ recieve   ✓ receive
2. ___ definately   ✓ definitely   8. ___ pnumonia   ✓ pneumonia
3. ✓ dining   ___ dinning   9. ___ rotator cup   ✓ rotator cuff
4. ___ excercise   ✓ exercise   10. ___ tolorate   ✓ tolerate
5. ___ parrafin   ✓ paraffin   11 ___ therapy puddy ✓ therapy putty
6. ___ transfering   ✓ transferring   12 ✓ independent   ___ independant

Worksheet 5-3: Spelling—More Practice

Place a check mark next to the word that is spelled correctly.
1. ✓ counseling   ___ counselling
2. ✓ diarrhea   ___ diarrea
3. ___ hemhorrage   ✓ hemorrhage
4. ✓ benefit   ___ benifit
5. ✓ interfered   ___ interferred
6. ___ eyesite   ✓ eyesight
7. ___ pullies   ✓ pulleys
8. ___ extention   ✓ extension
9. ___ hygeine   ✓ hygiene
10. ✓ preparation   ___ preperation
11. ✓ therapeutic   ___ theraputic
12. ___ flexability ✓ flexibility
13. ✓ strength   ___ strenth
14. ___ assymetrical ✓ asymmetrical
15. ✓ toilet   ___ toilet
16. ✓ leisure   ___ liesure
17. ✓ nauseous   ___ nauseus

Worksheet 5-4: Using Words Correctly

1. The home health *aide* gave the patient a shower.
2. The client refused to *accept* the doctor's diagnosis.
3. The traumatic brain injury will have a tremendous *effect* on activities of daily living.
4. If the client falls, she probably will *break* her hip due to osteoporosis.
5. The patient became short of *breath* after ambulating to the bathroom.
6. The client stated she wanted to *lose* ten pounds.

7. The patient injured her *dominant* right hand, which prevented her from writing.
8. The occupational therapy room is *farther* down the hallway than the physical therapy room.
9. The *current* caseload consists of 10 clients, as compared to 15 clients last week.
10. The OTR asked the patient to *lay* the scissors down on the table.
11. The weight of the pan was more *than* the patient could manage.
12. The clients in the craft group put *their* projects away in the closet.
13. The child was able to remain quiet and *stationary* while standing in line.
14. The *principal* of the school attended the IEP meeting.

Worksheet 5-5: Using Words Correctly—More Practice

1. The client has difficulty *gripping* the steering wheel.
2. The client was able to navigate his wheelchair throughout the store's *aisles* without knocking anything over.
3. The patient refused to take *personal* responsibility for his actions.
4. The patient reported pain when his biceps muscle was *palpated* by the OTA.
5. The client was able to *perform* all bathing tasks without assistance.
6. The child asked for a *piece* of candy.
7. The client had difficulty swallowing liquids due to *dysphagia*.
8. The student was denied *access* to the client's medical record.
9. The client followed the OTA's *advice* and purchased a shower chair.
10. A buttonhook can be a useful assistive *device* for clients with impaired dexterity.
11. The student was *adept* at playing the violin.
12. The client developed a lung infection due to *aspiration* of food.
13. The resident was very *impulsive* during transfers as she would not wait for the wheelchair to be properly positioned and locked before trying to stand up.

Mini Worksheet 5-6: Capitals

1. The OTA put the chart on the Occupational Therapist's desk.
2. The Patient was going to see his Doctor this afternoon.
3. The OT Aide used velcro and Scotch Tape to fix Mrs. Smith's lapboard during the occupational therapy session.
4. The Doctor spoke to the child who has Chicken Pox.
5. The OTA Student performed a Sensory Test on the client.
6. The client took Tylenol and Antacids before his Business Meeting.
7. The Nurse told the new mother that the infant has down syndrome.
8. The Physical Therapist informed the OTA that their client was admitted to the Hospital due to Pneumonia.
9. The Occupational therapy assistant worked in the outpatient department.
10. The OT used the Miller assessment for preschoolers to assess the child with Autism.

Mini Worksheet 5-7: Pronouns, Plurals, Possessives

Look at the following sentences and determine the incorrect components in each sentence. The corrections are provided in bold.
1. The three *clients'* appointments were all canceled today because their OTA was ill.
2. The *OTA's* lab coat was new.
3. The OTA *student's* resumé was reviewed by the OT. –or- The OTA *student's* resumé was reviewed by *his* OT. –or- The OTA *student's* resumé was reviewed by *her* OT.

Worksheet 8-2: Being Specific About Assist Levels

Without having seen the treatment session, it is impossible to know what part of the tasks required assistance. Here are some suggestions for how the statement might have been worded:

1.   Client supine → sit with min (A); bed → w/c with mod (A).

    Client supine → sit with min (A) to initiate activity; bed → w/c with mod (A) for balance.

    Client supine → sit with min (A) to pull up using trapeze; bed → w/c with mod (A) to lift body weight.

    Client supine → sit with min (A) to sequence movement; bed → w/c with mod (A) to bring body to 45°.

    Client supine → sit with min (A) swinging legs to EOB; bed → w/c with mod (A) for postural control.

2.   Client required SBA in transferring w/c ↔ toilet.

    Client required SBA for proper hand placement in transferring w/c ↔ toilet.

    Client required SBA to remind him of steps of the transfer when transferring w/c ↔ toilet.

    Client required SBA to remind him to lock w/c brakes and lean forward in order to rise from chair when transferring w/c ↔ toilet.

3.   Client retrieved garments from low drawers with min (A).

    Client retrieved garments from low drawers with min (A) to open drawers.

    Client retrieved garments from low drawers with min (A) to release trigger on reacher.

    Client retrieved garments from low drawers with min (A) to judge halo placement in space.

    Client retrieved garments from low drawers with min (A) to grasp handles of drawers.

4.   Brushing hair required max (A).

    Brushing hair required max (A) to hold brush.

    Brushing hair required max (A) to reach back of head.

    Brushing hair required max (A) to flex shoulder past 35°.

5.   Client completed dressing, toileting, and hygiene with min (A).

    Client completed dressing, toileting, and hygiene with min (A) for sitting balance.

    Client completed dressing, toileting, and hygiene with min (A) to reach feet.

    Client completed dressing, toileting, and hygiene with min (A) for activities requiring fine motor dexterity.

    Client completed dressing, toileting, and hygiene with min (A) to adhere to hip precautions.

Chapter 9

Worksheet 9-1: Justifying Continued Treatment

Which of the following require the skill of an OTA?

1.   *No*   Administering paraffin irrelevant to occupational performance

2.   *Yes*   Instructing the client in leisure skills for stress management

3.   *No*   Having a client watch a video on assertiveness training without further instruction or without role-playing the techniques

4.   *Yes*   Analyzing and modifying functional tasks/activities through the provision of adaptive equipment, or techniques

5.   *Yes*   Determining that the modified task is safe and effective

6.   *No*   Carrying out a maintenance program

7.   *Yes*   Upgrading a strengthening program

8.   *Yes*   Teaching the client to use the breathing techniques he has learned while performing his ADL activities

9.   *No*   Interpreting initial evaluation results and establishing the intervention plan *(this is the responsibility of the OT)*

10. *Yes* Providing individualized instruction to the client, family, or caregiver
11. *No* Giving the patient a replacement piece of hook and loop fastener
12. *Yes* Providing specialized instruction to eliminate limitations in a functional activity
13. *Yes* Developing a home program and instructing caregivers
14. *Yes* Teaching compensatory skills
15. *No* Gait training
16. *Yes* Making skilled recommendations to a parent for a child's positioning and feeding
17. *Yes* Educating clients to eliminate safety hazards
18. *No* Presenting information handouts (such as energy conservation) without having the client perform the activity
19. *No* Routine exercise and strengthening programs
20. *Yes* Adding instruction in lower body dressing techniques to a current ADL program
21. *Yes* Teaching adaptive techniques such as one-handed shoe tying
22. *No* Helping a client in the bathroom *(an aide or family member can help a client; OTAs provide skilled instruction or modification of the task)*
23. *No* Asking a client about his day *(skilled occupational therapy is assessing information pertinent to the intervention plan, not just conversing with a client)*

Mini Worksheet 9-2: Organizing Your Thoughts for Assessment

Problems
Safety of transferring to and from the toilet

Client factors that were not WFL (AROM shoulder abduction).

Decreased performance skills (activity tolerance and dynamic balance)

Progress/potential
Verbalized an understanding of safety instructions

PROM ®̄ shoulder abduction WNL

Worksheet 9-3: Assessing Factors Not Within Functional Limits

1. Child wrote poorly due to immature pencil grasp and difficulty c̄ spatial orientation of letters.
    Poor visual-spatial perception and immature pencil grasp interfere with writing skills.

2. Client demonstrated difficulty with balancing her checkbook due to memory and sequencing deficits.
    Memory and sequencing deficits cause difficulty c̄ IADL tasks such as balancing checkbook.

3. Client experiencing manic episode and was unable to attend and follow directions for cooking activity.
    Client's ↓ process skills 2° manic episode limit performance of cooking and other IADL tasks.

4. Client problem solved poorly while performing lower body dressing as evidenced by multiple attempts to button pants and don socks.
    Client's ↓ ability to problem solve limits her ability to dress herself without Ⓐ and raises safety concerns in all ADL areas.

Worksheet 9-4: Social Skills Worksheet

What **problems** do you see in the above "S" and "O"?
Unkempt appearance

Interrupts others when talking

Does not stay on topic of conversation

What **areas of occupation** do these problems impact?
Social participation

What evidence of **progress** and/or **potential** do you see?

Engages in conversation

States that she understands the purpose of the group

Willingness to participate in the group

Spontaneously shared her ideas and experiences

A: *Client's unkempt appearance, interrupting behaviors, and need for redirection to topic of conversation inter-fere with her ability to engage in social participation with peers. Her expressed interest in groups and her willingness to engage in conversation and share her ideas show good potential to develop relationships and to express herself verbally in place of acting out. Client would benefit from participating in groups where conver-sational skills are stressed along with further facilitation of attention to social cues, and from assistance with ADL activities stressing hygiene and appearance.*

Chapter 10

Mini Worksheet 10-1: Determining the Plan

P: *Continue OT 5X wk for 1 week for skilled instruction in safe transfers and toileting. Home program for AROM and strengthening exercises for Ⓡ shoulder will be taught.*

-or-

P: *Continue OT for 1 hour 5 X wk for 1 week to work on safe transfers, toileting, and improving activity tolerance. Client will be instructed in HEP to improve Ⓡ shoulder AROM and strength.*

Worksheet 10-2: Completing the Social Skills Plan

P: *Client to continue daily OT for the next week to ↑ interpersonal skills and BADLs needed for social participa-tion in a variety of contexts.*

-or-

P: *Client to continue social skills group 3 X wk and to be given individual feedback daily on her attention to appearance and social cues.*

Worksheet 10-3: Completing the Plan—Additional Practice

P: *Client to continue OT 2 X wk to ↑ Ⓡ hand strength, functional fine motor skills, and BADLs. Next session, client will be instructed in one-handed shoe tying technique and will be assessed for return demonstration of HEP.*

-or-

P: *Client to continue OT twice weekly for instruction in compensatory techniques and remediation of Ⓡ fine motor skills and hand strength to enable BADL performance. Client will be instructed in adaptive equipment in order to manage all clothing fastenings Ⓘ. HEP to be upgraded by increasing resistance of therapy putty next week.*

Chapter 12

Worksheet 12-1: Mechanics of Documentation

1. Time of day not recorded
2. No health record number or identification number present
3. Last name is not listed first (may not be required by facility to list last name first)
4. Spaces present without line drawn

5. Error not corrected properly—should have date and initials above or next to the error
6. No cosignature (will depend on facility and legal guidelines)
7. Type of note not indicated (contact note)
8. Occupational therapy department not indicated
9. Spelling error (deferred)
10. OTA's first name only indicated by initial

Worksheet 12-2: Documentation Basics

For each of the following SOAP note sentences, correct any errors in spelling, grammar, abbreviations, and basic mechanics of documentation.

1. The client used **compensitory** techniques to **donn** his shoes and socks.

   The client used compensatory techniques to don his shoes and socks.

2. The client performed bed mobility Ⓘ, then sat on **SOB** with SBA to doff his shirt.

   The client performed bed mobility Ⓘ, then sat on EOB with SBA to doff his shirt.

   (SOB is the abbreviation for shortness of breath.)

3. Child **was seen** for 20 minutes in classroom **to help** her put her coat on.

   Child participated in 20-minute session in classroom to improve skills needed for donning her coat.

   -or-

   Child participated in 20-minute session in classroom for skilled BADL instruction.

   (Remember to show active client participation in therapy. Also, as a teacher or aide could help the child put a coat on, be sure to indicate the skilled services that the occupational therapy practitioner is providing.)

4. Client stated he will "not wear **his** splint to work."

   Client stated he will not wear his splint to work.

   -or-

   Client stated, "I will not wear my splint to work."

5. The **CVA pt.** demonstrated ability to transfer bed ↔ commode with SBA and **VC**.

   The pt. diagnosed with CVA demonstrated ability to transfer bed ↔ commode with SBA and verbal cues.

   or-

   The pt. who sustained a CVA demonstrated ability to transfer bed ↔ commode with SBA and verbal cues.

   (Remember to use people-first language. Also, VC is the abbreviation for vital capacity.)

6. The child demonstrated progress by using her **bad** hand to stabilize the paper when writing.

   The child demonstrated progress by using her affected hand (or involved hand or weak hand) to stabilize the paper when writing.

   (Don't use "bad" or "good" to delineate limbs.)

7. During her **Occupational Therapy** session, the pt. worked on ↑ Ⓛ neglect and ↓ safety to perform ADLs.

   During her occupational therapy session, the pt. worked on therapeutic activities to ↓ Ⓛ neglect and ↑ safety to perform ADLs.

   -or-

   During her occupational therapy session, the pt. worked on increasing awareness of Ⓛ side and improving safety during ADLs.

   (In the incorrect example, it seems to indicate that therapy is working to increase the client's neglect and decrease her safety rather than what is intended.)

8. **I** instructed the client in **arom** exercises to improve her ability to braid her two **daughter's** hair.

   Client was instructed in AROM exercises to improve her ability to braid her two daughters' hair.

   (Focus on the client and not the practitioner.)

9. The client performed self-feeding with **modified assistance**.

    The client performed self-feeding with modified independence.

    -or-

    The client performed self-feeding with moderate assistance.

    (Modified assistance is not a standard term.)

10. The **THR client's** (L) hip is sore because **the PT made her walk too long**.

    The client with a (L) THR reported (L) hip soreness following PT session.

    -or-

    The client who had (L) hip replacement surgery reported soreness in (L) hip after ambulating in PT.

    (Use people-first language and do not make subjective or judgmental statements about another professional in your note.)

11. The student **was** mod assist to write her name.

    The student needed mod assist to write her name due to difficulty holding pencil 2° spasticity.

    -or-

    The student required mod assist to write her name due to difficulty with spatial orientation of letters.

    -or-

    The student required mod assist to write her name due to poor task attention.

    (Indicate that the client needs assist rather than the client is an assist level. Also, describe what part of the task needed assistance.)

Chapter 13

Worksheet 13-1: SOAPing Your Note

1. *O* Client supine → sit in bed (I).
2. *O* Client moved kitchen items from counter to cabinet (I) using (L) hand.
3. *S* Parent reports child's handwriting has significantly improved within the past month.
4. *A* Problems include decreased coordination, strength, sensation, and proprioception in left hand, which create safety risks in home management tasks.
5. *S* Client reports that his fingers are stiff this morning and that he is having trouble handling small items like buttons.
6. *P* By the end of next treatment session, client will demonstrate ability to don/doff splint (I).
7. *A* Increase of 15 minutes in activity tolerance for UE activities permits her to prepare a light meal (I).
8. *O* Child participated in 30-minute OT session to promote development of FM skills for BADLs.
9. *A* Deficits in proprioception and motor planning limit client's ability to dress herself.
10. *P* Continue ROM and retrograde massage to (R) hand for edema control and to enable grasp of objects needed for BADLs.
11. *P* Consumer will be seen 2X weekly to improve attention to task in order to obtain a job.
12. *S* Client reports that she cannot remember her hip precautions.
13. *A* Client would benefit from further instruction to incorporate total hip precautions into lower body dressing, bathing, and toilet hygiene.
14. *A* Learning was evident by client's ability to improve with repetition.

15. *A*   Client's request to take rest breaks demonstrates knowledge of her limitations in endurance.

16. *O*   Client required three verbal prompts to interact with peers in OT social group.

17. *A*   Fair+ muscle grade of extension in Ⓡ wrist extensors this week shows good progress toward goals.

18. *A*   Poor temporal organization interferes with getting to work on time.

19. *P*   Next session, instruct parent in proper positioning of infant for bottle feeding.

20. *O*   Client demonstrated ability to perform sliding board transfer w/c ↔ mat with min assist to position board properly.

Worksheet 13-2: Writing the "S"—Subjective

S: *Client reported significant arthritis in Ⓡ shoulder and Ⓡ knee, and a preference to approach transfers from the affected side. Client stated it hurts to bear weight on her Ⓡ leg and reported pain as 7/10. She also stated w/c → bed sliding board transfers are the most difficult, and reported fatigue after transfer.*

-or-

S: *Client reported arthritis in Ⓡ shoulder and Ⓡ knee and stated knee pain is 7/10 when bearing weight on Ⓡ LE. Pt. able to verbalize needs regarding transfer (placement of board and approach from affected side). Client reported fatigue after transfer.*

Worksheet 13-3: Making Opening Lines Better

1.   Client practiced laundry tasks for 45 minutes.

   Client participated in 45-minute session in her room to increase Ⓘ in IADLs, to decrease safety concerns during functional mobility, and to provide instruction on proper use of adaptive equipment for home management tasks.

   -or-

   Client participated in OT 45 minutes in hospital room for skilled instruction on use of adaptive equipment to safely perform home management tasks.

   -or-

   In hospital room, client participated in 45-minute session for education on safety concerns during IADLs and skilled instruction in use of adaptive equipment for laundry tasks.

   -or-

   In OT clinic, client participated in 45-minute session for education in use of adaptive equipment and hip precautions during performance of home management tasks.

2.   Consumer seen at workshop for 1 hour to improve job skills.

   At workshop, consumer participated in 1-hour session to address time management, cognitive, sensory, and bilateral integration barriers to performing work tasks effectively.

   -or-

   Consumer participated in OT for 1 hr. at workshop to work on sequencing, bilateral coordination, concentration, and time management skills while completing work task of package handling.

   -or-

   In order to improve time management and sequencing skills, increase bilateral coordination, and decrease distractibility for package handling at work, consumer participated in 60-minute OT session at workshop.

   -or-

   Consumer participated in 1-hr. session at workshop for skilled instruction in task sequencing, bilateral coordination, and techniques to improve time management and decrease distractibility for job skills.

3. Client seen in his hospital room bedside for 30 minutes for feeding.

    Client participated in 30-minute session bedside for instruction in adaptive equipment for feeding and perceptual remediation.

    -or-

    Client participated in 30-minute session bedside to increase Ⓘ self-feeding and to decrease Ⓛ neglect.

    -or-

    Client participated in 30-minute session bedside for education in compensatory methods for feeding and to ↑ awareness of left side.

    -or-

    At bedside for 30 minutes, client participated in OT for skilled instruction in self-feeding methods and to improve perceptual skills.

4. Worked with client in kitchen for 1 hr. to ↑ Ⓘ in cooking.

    Client participated in 1-hr. session in OT kitchen to increase activity tolerance for standing and increase awareness of affected UE for safety in cooking.

    -or-

    In OT kitchen, client participated in 1-hr. session to address safety concerns regarding standing tolerance and Ⓛ UE neglect.

    -or-

    Client participated in 60-minute OT session in kitchen to work on cooking tasks with attention to standing tolerance, affected UE position, and safety.

    -or-

    In OT kitchen, client participated in 1-hr. session for skilled IADL instruction to improve safety, standing tolerance, and attention to affected UE.

Worksheet 13-4: Writing the "O"—Objective

- First an opening line is needed stating where, for how long, and for what purpose the client was seen. One possibility is:

    Client participated in 45-minute OT session in room for skilled instruction in BADL tasks and assessment of splinting needs.

    -or-

    Client participated in 60-minute session bedside for skilled instruction in compensatory techniques for dressing, toilet hygiene, and assessment of splinting needs.

- Second, the categories could be reduced to three (toileting, dressing, and splinting assessment) or two (BADLs and splinting assessment), and the statements about donning shoes can be combined.

- Third, different assist levels are listed for upper body dressing, which is confusing. It would be helpful to know what parts of the task needed what kind of assistance. Also, more information about the type of toilet transfer would be useful. Did the client transfer from a w/c? Was a sliding board, walker, or grab bars used?

- Fourth, the UE and LE wording is not inclusive enough because the client is dressing the upper and lower body rather than just the extremities. Specific types of clothing are not indicated (i.e., elastic waist paints, turtleneck sweater). The note also does not indicate where the client got dressed. Was the client sitting on the edge of the bed, in a w/c, or in a chair?

- Finally, under hand status, there is no functional component, and "index finger greatest amount" is not very informative.

Worksheet 13-5: Differentiating Between Observations and Assessments

1. *O* Client is unable to don Ⓛ LE prosthesis for functional mobility.

2. *A* Inability to don Ⓛ LE prosthesis Ⓘ prevents client from performing safe functional mobility around the house to live alone.

3. *A* Decreased tolerance to auditory stimuli limits the student's ability to attend to classroom tasks.

4. *O* Student required three verbal cues to stay on task due to decreased tolerance to auditory stimuli.

5. *O* Client was unable to incorporate relaxation and stress reduction techniques, requiring several verbal prompts to complete task.

6. *A* Inability to incorporate relaxation and stress reduction techniques when interacting with sales clerk limits her ability to manage shopping tasks Ⓘ after discharge.

1. Client demonstrated difficulty with balancing checkbook due to memory and sequencing deficits.

   Decreased memory and sequencing abilities limit client's ability to perform IADLs such as financial management tasks.

   -or-

   Memory and sequencing deficits interfere with client's ability to perform IADLs such as financial management tasks, and limit her ability to return to an Ⓘ living situation.

   -or-

   Deficits in memory and sequencing limit the client's ability to do many IADLs, for example, balancing her checkbook.

   -or-

   Deficits in memory and sequencing lead to difficulty with IADLs such as financial management tasks necessary for household management.

2. Client unable to complete homemaking tasks or basic self-care activities independently due to Ⓛ neglect, impulsive behavior, and decreased attention to task.

   Decreased safety awareness, poor attention, and perceptual deficits limit client's ability to complete homemaking tasks and self-care activities Ⓘ.

   -or-

   Decreased safety awareness and inattention to Ⓛ side interfere with client's ability to complete homemaking tasks and decrease her ability to successfully complete basic activities of daily living Ⓘ.

   -or-

   Decreased safety awareness and cognitive/perceptual deficits prevent client from performing homemaking and BADLs Ⓘ and safely.

3. After the use of behavior modification techniques, child demonstrated ability to remain seated at his desk for the remainder of the treatment session.

   You could take a positive or a negative approach to this one.

   Positive:
   Child's ability to remain seated at desk with the aid of behavior modification techniques indicates good potential for improving problem behaviors in school.

   -or-

   Child's positive response to behavior modification techniques shows good potential to meet classroom behavior goals.

   Negative:
   The need for behavior modification techniques to remain seated at desk limit child's ability to succeed with academic tasks.

   -or-

   Child's need for behavior modification in order to remain seated limits his ability to concentrate effectively in classroom situations.

Worksheet 13-6: Problems, Progress, and Rehab Potential

Problems:

After reading through this note, several problems stood out for this OTA:

- Dynamic sitting balance
- Weight shifting
- Posture
- Transfers

The four above are related to safety and functional mobility.

- Decreased AROM in Ⓡ UE (mod Ⓐ to reach)
- Cognition

On thinking a little further, the OTA decided that the "cognition" problem might really be one of the following because the client does seem to understand the goal of the activity.

- Short-term memory
- Motor planning
- Problem solving
- Initiation

Finally, the OTA decides that the problem with initiation is probably some combination of problem-solving and motor planning deficit.

Progress/Rehab Potential

- Ability to understand the treatment goal

The OTA then groups the problems according to the impact they have on the client's occupational performance. The OTA decides that the first three cause difficulty with functional mobility and are of particular concern because they create safety issues. The motor planning and initiation problem is a concern in the area of self-care, as is the problem with decreased AROM of the right UE. The need for continual instruction, whether it is a problem with short-term memory or with his ability to problem solve, is likely to require a lot of attention from a caregiver at home. The client does, however, understand why he is doing the given task. As long as the goals are not set too high, the client should be able to make good progress in rehabilitation. The OTA's assessment and plan read as follows:

A: *Deficits in postural control, dynamic sitting balance, and weight shifting raise safety concerns when transferring. ↓ AROM and motor planning ability negatively impact ability to perform self-care tasks. A need for continual instruction to prevent unsafe performance of ADL tasks requires a high level of caregiver assistance. Client's ability to understand treatment goal indicates good rehab potential for the goals established. Client would benefit from continued skilled instruction in activities to ↑ balance, safe functional mobility, and facilitate Ⓘ in ADL tasks.*

P: *Continue OT daily for 3 weeks for skilled instruction in self-care tasks and safe transfers. Next session, instruct client in w/c ↔ toilet transfer using grab bar to facilitate forward weight shifting in w/c.*

Another OTA might assess the session a little differently. For example:

A: *Problems include deficits in motor planning, movement initiation, cognition, and muscle weakness in Ⓡ UE, which ↓ safety in ADL tasks and functional mobility. Activity tolerance for Ⓡ UE reaching tasks has improved since yesterday from <1 minute to >3 minutes without a rest break. Client would benefit from skilled OT to increase balance, functional mobility, and grasp/release activities with involved UE in order to ↑ Ⓘ in self-care activities.*

P: *Continue OT twice daily for half-hour sessions to work on Ⓡ UE movement and cognitive retraining in order to complete grooming activities with min Ⓐ. Next session will focus on facilitating Ⓡ hand grasp for grooming, such as squeezing toothpaste tube and holding hairbrush.*

-or-

A: *Decreased functional use of the (R) UE, decreased sitting balance, and difficulty with sequencing and problem solving limit ability to perform ADLs. Increased shoulder flexion and improved motor planning since initial evaluation, and increased understanding of treatment activities indicate good rehab potential. Client would benefit from continued skilled OT for exercises to increase functional AROM, grasp, and weight shifting to improve dynamic sitting balance. Client would also benefit from evaluation of both cognitive status and ability to initiate activity in order to increase (I) in ADL tasks.*

P: *Continue OT twice daily for 30-minute sessions for 2 weeks to increase dynamic sitting balance in preparation for ADLs. Client will be able to reach for grooming items placed slightly beyond arm's reach with CGA within 1 week.*

Worksheet 13-7: The "Almost" Note

Here we have a note that seems good on the surface, but it demonstrates some problems in critical thinking and organization. The most outstanding problem with this note is that the OTA is mixing the "O" data and the "A" data.

First, it would have helped the "S" if the OTA had asked pertinent questions, such as what the client's pain levels were.

Second, the note should indicate active client participation rather than the client just being "seen" in therapy. There is nothing in the "O" to show that skilled occupational therapy is being provided. The list of observations of assist levels fails to provide the richness of the skill used in treatment. The OTA erroneously puts some of that information in the "A" section, rather than assessing the data. In the "A" the OTA tells us:

Deficits noted in (R) UE coordination, (B) UE strength, and dynamic standing balance. Client (I) in dressing EOB, but is min (A) in dressing when standing with a walker. (L) UE AROM is WFL but (R) UE has deficits noted in shoulder flexion. Client needs SBA in bed mobility when rolling to unaffected side and min (A) in sit → stand 2° ↓ UE strength. Client needs SBA for transfer to unaffected side in pivot transfer bed → w/c and min (A) w/c → toilet. Client would benefit from skilled OT to continue UE strengthening and coordination exercises and to ↑ dynamic standing balance using walker, in order to ↑ (I) in ADLs.

Even if this information were moved into the "O," there is nothing to tell us what part of the task the assistance was for. The OTA uses a nonstandard abbreviation "VCs." The OTA means verbal cues, but since VC is a standard health term meaning *vital capacity*, it is inappropriate in its usage here and is not on the "approved" list in this manual. Also, the OTA should be more specific than simply stating, "↓ *range in shoulder flexion*." For example, is shoulder flexion 90 degrees or 150 degrees? Does the ROM deficit limit ability to dress or use walker?

Third, the coordination deficits mentioned in the "A" section come out of the blue. There is no mention of coordination in the opening statement "...*for work on dressing and functional mobility*," nor is it mentioned as a problem in the "O." Thus, the statement that coordination deficits are one of the problems noted and the statement that the client would benefit from coordination exercises are unsubstantiated. Remember not to introduce any new information in the "A" section of your note. Information regarding transfers and bed mobility is redundant because it is simply stated twice without any additional assessment or clinical judgment. Also, do not state that the client *is* an assist level but, instead, *needs* the assist level

There is no real assessment of the meaning of the data found in the "S" and the "O." There is a short list of problem areas, but no assessment of their impact on the ability to engage in meaningful occupation, and no assessment of the rehab potential shown by the client's willingness to "do whatever it takes to get out of the hospital."

The best thing for this OTA to do is to rewrite the "O" section, providing a more comprehensive picture of the treatment session. Then, the OTA needs to assess the data based on skilled observations and clinical reasoning. There needs to be an indication of how the observed data impacts the occupational performance of the client before the statements about what the client would benefit from.

Depending on the assessment the OTA makes, the plan to work on balance may be appropriate, or it may be only one of the things to be addressed. The note does not indicate if the client's deficits are due to cognitive problems such as memory deficits, poor problem solving, or decreased safety awareness. Does the client have limited endurance or poor motor planning? Those might be additional areas that need to be addressed in the plan. Also, the client may benefit from further occupational therapy to work on safe transfers, and further retraining in dressing or other BADLs.

Chapter 14

Worksheet 14-1: Initial Evaluation Report

Background Data

Criteria	How Does the Evaluation Comply With the Criteria?
Are all of the following present: name, date of birth, gender? Are all applicable diagnoses listed?	*Name, date of birth, and gender are all indicated.* *Dx: CVA; R/O OBS* *2° Dx: Type 2 diabetes*
Is it clear who referred the client to OT, on what date, and what services were requested?	*Dr. Heelue referred her for evaluation and treatment on 5/3/2012.*
Is the funding source listed for this client?	*Medicare*
Is anticipated length of stay indicated for this client?	*2 weeks*
Why is the client seeking occupational therapy services?	*She wants to be independent and return home.*
Are there any secondary problems, preexisting conditions, contraindications or precautions that will impact therapy?	*Diabetes*

Occupational History and Profile

Is there an occupational history/profile? Is it adequate?	*There is a brief occupational profile. More information can be obtained during tx.*
Which areas of occupation are currently successful and which are problematic?	*No successful areas noted. ADL and IADL tasks are problematic.*
What factors hinder the client's performance in areas of occupation? What factors support performance in areas of occupation?	***Hinder***: ↓ *problem-solving ability, slow cognitive responses* ↓ *ability to initiate and sequence tasks. Some client factors not WNL.* ***Support***: *A nearby daughter who is willing to visit daily and assist with transportation, intact sensation, motor planning and perception WFL, able to stand and transfer with CGA, one-story home, sedentary hobbies, motivation to go home.*
What are the client's priorities? What does the client hope to gain from OT?	*To be Ⓘ and go back to her own home*
What areas of occupation will be targeted for intervention? Do these match the client's priorities?	*ADLs and IADLs, which do match the client's priorities*
What are the targeted outcomes?	*Discharge to home* *Modified Ⓘ and safety in ADL activities*

Results of the Assessment

What types of assessments were used?	*Mini-Mental State, ADL evaluation, manual muscle test, sensation, observation, interview, AROM*
What were the results of the assessments?	*Results are clearly noted on the evaluation form and in the "A."*
What client factors, contextual aspects and activity demands are identified as needing attention?	***Client factors***: ↓ *AROM and strength in the Ⓛ UE,* ↓ *activity tolerance,* ↓ *problem solving, sequencing, and memory* ***Context***: *lives alone and daughter unable to provide supervision; needs cues for orientation.* ***Activity demands***: *Needs cues to initiate and sequence activities and to problem solve.*

What factors (strengths, supports) facilitate the client's occupational performance?	*Supportive daughter, client motivated to be* Ⓘ
Are there other areas that need to be assessed that are not listed?	*Does client use hearing aid, glasses, or ambulation devices? Does client have pain, edema, or changes in muscle tone? Other considerations for occupational profile (e.g., spiritual or virtual contexts? educational level? habits and routines?)*
Is OT appropriate for this client? Why or why not?	*Yes—client has good rehab potential to return home and requires OT to improve ADL function and safety.*

Worksheet 14-2: Intervention Plan

Criteria	How Does The Evaluation Comply With the Criteria?
Are specific occupational therapy interventions identified?	*Yes*
Are the intervention goals and objectives measurable and realistic?	*Yes*
Are the goals and objectives directly related to the client's occupational role performance?	*Yes*
What is the anticipated frequency/duration of services?	*45-minute sessions 5X wk for 2 weeks*
What is the discontinuation criteria or expected outcomes?	*Ability to live at home safely without supervision*
What is the anticipated discharge location?	*Home*
What is the anticipated plan for follow-up care?	*Meeting with daughter*
Where will service be provided?	*Healthy Hospital as inpatient*

Mini Worksheet 14-4: Choosing Activities—More Practice

How could you work on these goals at the same time? What would your treatment activities be?

1. *Student will be able to open all containers and wrappers* Ⓘ *for his lunch at school*
2. *In order to perform bimanual classroom tasks, student will use* Ⓛ *hand spontaneously as a functional assist 5/5 opportunities.*
3. *Student will attend to classroom tasks for 10-minute periods with only one verbal cue for redirection.*

You can work with the child at lunchtime in the cafeteria or in another room. You could have the child try to open all of the lunch items such as lunch box, brown bag, milk carton, sandwich wrapper, straw wrapper, plastic containers, snack bags, etc. You will note if the child is incorporating use of both hands spontaneously for these tasks and how well the Ⓛ hand is being used as a functional assist for setting up lunch items. You will also note the number of minutes for attention to task and if child needs to be redirected to task.

-or-

You might also have the child perform another task that involves opening containers, such as a craft project where materials are in snack bags or small jars/containers. Again, you would note Ⓛ hand use and attention span.

Chapter 15

Worksheet 15-1: Evaluating Goal Statements

1. By the time of discharge in 1 week, client will be able to dress himself with min Ⓐ for balance using a sock aid and reacher while sitting in a wheelchair.

   This goal has all the necessary COAST components to be useful.

2. Client will tolerate 15 minutes of treatment daily.

   This goal lacks a function and a time frame. In addition, the behavior (tolerating treatment) is not useful because it is not something a client needs to do after discharge. This would be better stated as "tolerate 15 minutes of grooming/hygiene activity."

3. Client will demonstrate increased coping skills in order to live at home with her granddaughter within 2 weeks.

   This goal lacks specificity, and it needs a condition. "Coping skills" is far too broad. The coping skill(s) in question need to be specified.

4. Resident will demonstrate 15 minutes of activity tolerance without rest breaks using Ⓑ UE in order to complete self-care tasks before breakfast each morning.

   This goal lacks a time frame and needs to be turned around to put function first. For example: Resident will be able to complete BADLs in <15 minutes without rest breaks before breakfast each morning within 2 weeks.

5. In order to be able to toilet self after discharge, client will demonstrate ability to perform a sliding board transfer w/c → mat within the next week.

   This goal has all the necessary COAST components to be useful but would be even better if the assist level of the transfer were noted (e.g., modified Ⓘ).

6. OTA will teach lower body dressing using a reacher, dressing stick, and sock aid within 2 treatment sessions.

   This goal lacks a proper client action and behavior and should focus on what the client, not the OT or OTA, will do.

7. In order to return to living independently, client will demonstrate ability to balance his checkbook.

   This goal lacks a time frame and would be even better if the assist level for balancing his checkbook were specified (e.g., ability to balance his checkbook Ⓘ).

Worksheet 15-2: Writing Goals That Are Client-Centered, Occupation-Based, and Measurable

Without knowing the client, it is impossible to know what the goal would really be. Here are some suggestions.

1. *Within three treatment sessions, client will complete a cooking activity with supervision and maintain task attention >10 minutes without redirection.*

   -or-

   Client will demonstrate 10-minute attention span for cooking, requiring no more than 3 verbal cues for redirection by the end of the 3rd treatment session.

2. *By anticipated discharge in 1 week, client will cook a packaged microwave meal with min Ⓐ to follow three-step written directions.*

   -or-

   Client will demonstrate ability to follow a three-step recipe Ⓘ within 1 week.

3. *Client will be able to don shirt with modified Ⓘ using the over-the-head method and a buttonhook within two treatment sessions.*

   -or-

   Client will be able to dress upper body with modified Ⓘ using one-handed techniques and adaptive equipment within 1 week.

4. *By discharge in 2 weeks, client will demonstrate ability to complete simulated childcare bathing and diapering tasks, standing at least 10 minutes Ⓘ without rest breaks.*

   -or-

   Client will complete seated work-simulation tasks (filing and data entry) for 30 minutes without rest breaks within 1 week.

5. *Client will make change from $1.00 correctly 3/3 tries within 2 weeks.*

   -or-

   Client will select ads from the newspaper for an apartment that rents for less than 1/3 of his regular monthly income with minimal verbal cues within the next month.

6. *Within 1 week, client will spontaneously complete showering, dressing, and grooming prior to attending morning groups 3/3 days.*

   -or-

   Client will verbalize an interest in at least one future activity without prompting within the next 2 days.

Worksheet 15-3: Writing Goals—Developmental Disability

Without knowing the client, it is impossible to know what the goals should really be. Here are some suggestions for functional goals:

1. **Instrumental ADL—meal preparation**: *Client will be able to wash and peel vegetables to make a salad with min verbal cues within 4 weeks.*

   -or-

   Client will prepare a one-step frozen breakfast item with supervision using toaster or microwave safely within 3 weeks.

2. **Instrumental ADL—household chore**: *Client will be able to follow the chore schedule for changing bed sheets with one verbal reminder within 4 weeks.*

   -or-

   Client will demonstrate ability to set the table Ⓘ for six place settings within 1 week.

3. **Instrumental ADL—shopping**: *Client will locate five items in supermarket using grocery list with 1 verbal cue for each item within 4 weeks.*

   -or-

   Client will be able to locate correct size clothing when shopping within 2 weeks.

4. **Instrumental ADL—money management/functional math skill**: *When shopping, client will use correct denominations to pay cashier Ⓘ for items up to $10.00 within 6 weeks.*

   -or-

   In order to improve shopping skills, client will select and place correct coins in vending machine Ⓘ within 3 weeks.

5. **Communication/interaction skills**: *Client will demonstrate improved social skills by cooperatively playing a simple board game with peers for 20 minutes within 3 weeks.*

   -or-

   Client will demonstrate improved interaction skills by spontaneously allowing roommate to choose TV program without an altercation within 3 weeks.

6. **Prevocational skills**: *To improve prevocational skills, client will demonstrate ability to correctly punch a time clock 5/5 opportunities within 2 weeks.*

   -or-

   In order to ↑ skills required for employment, client will select appropriate attire for job interview within 2 weeks.

7. **Temporal organization/time management**: *In order to improve time management skills for BADLs, client will set alarm clock with one verbal cue within 4 weeks.*

   -or-

   In order to improve time management skills for morning self-care, client will follow daily schedule Ⓘ within 1 week.

Worksheet 15-4: Goal Writing—Functional BADL Components

BADL: Brushing teeth
Goals will depend on a client's specific circumstances. However, here are some suggestions.

1. **Fine-motor skills**: *Client will demonstrate improved dexterity for grooming by demonstrating ability to open and close toothpaste cap Ⓘ within 2 weeks.*

   Within 3 treatment sessions, client will be able to use cylindrical grip to hold toothbrush with affected hand when applying toothpaste.

2. **Hand strength**: *Client will demonstrate improved hand strength for brushing teeth by holding 5-ounce cup of water with affected hand and bringing it to mouth Ⓘ within 1 week.*

   Child will demonstrate improved Ⓡ hand strength for grooming by squeezing toothpaste onto toothbrush with min Ⓐ within 1 week.

3. **Standing balance**: *When brushing teeth, child will demonstrate improved dynamic standing balance from poor to fair standing at sink with contact guard assist within 2 months.*

4. **Unilateral inattention**: *Client will demonstrate improved Ⓛ side attention for grooming by locating all items needed for tooth brushing with min verbal cues by 5/10/13.*

5. **Elbow range of motion**: *In order to facilitate tooth brushing, resident will increase Ⓡ elbow flexion by 30° by 3/19/13.*

6. **Problem solving**: *Client will demonstrate improved problem-solving skills for grooming by placing appropriate amount of toothpaste on brush within 1 week.*

7. **Spatial relations**: *Child will demonstrate improved spatial relations for grooming by applying toothpaste to brush Ⓘ without spilling within 1 wk.*

Chapter 17

Worksheet 17-1: Types of Documentation

1. *G. OASIS* — Outcome measure required by Medicare and Medicaid for use in home care

2. *F. IEP* — Yearly multidisciplinary plan established for a particular student requiring special services

3. *J. Intervention Plan* — Contains goals and specific treatment approaches relating to desired client outcomes

4. *D. Discontinuation Report* — Written when occupational therapy services are no longer needed

5. *B. Minimum Data Set* — Interdisciplinary assessment used in a skilled nursing facility to determine a client's problem areas and care plan

6. *H. Progress Report* — Summarizes course of treatment and progress toward achieving goals during specified intervals

7. *A. Contact Note* — Written following a treatment session and can include intervention provided, pertinent phone conversations, or meetings

8. *C. Initial Evaluation* — Consists of an occupational profile and factors affecting engagement in occupation

9. *I. Reevaluation Report* — A determination of the client's present status as compared to start of care, including progress, problems, and revision of goals

10. *K. Occupational Profile* — Includes the client's roles, responsibilities, and factors such as values, culture, physical and social environments, age, and educational level

11. *E. Transition Plan* — Written to provide consistency when a client switches from one setting to another during the treatment continuum

Index

supervision, appropriate, 28
symbols, in health record, 20, 31-40, 196-197

terminal illness, documentation for, 177
terminology, for recipients of service, 20
therapy cap, 28
therapy log, in contact notes, 156
time frames, in plan section, 91
timed services, 28
timeline, in COAST format, 145
transfers, documentation of, 75
transition plans, 8, 126
trauma, multiple, discharge note for, 184
treatment
    activities for, choosing, 138-139
    interruptions of, 96
    justification of continuation, 82-84, 204-205
    stages of, reports for, 155-164
    types of, notes for, 179
treatment media, de-emphasizing, 70-71, 203
    worksheet for, 72, 203
treatment notes. *See* contact (treatment) notes
treatment time, billing for, 24, 28
TRICARE, 26
truth, in documentation, 20

untimed services, 28
utilization record management, health record use in, 27-29

values, 4
verb tenses, in health record, 51
verification, of effective treatment, 80
video training aids, 12, 111
visit notes. *See* contact (treatment) notes

Weed, Lawrence, 15-16
wheelchair mobility, contact notes for, 190
work
    goal statements for, 148
    as treatment goal, 5
Worker's Compensation, 5
    funding from, 26
    health record for, 18
World Health Organization
    ICD codes of, 29
    International Classification of Functioning, Disability and Health (ICF), 3

A Quick Checklist for Evaluating Your Note

Use the following two summary charts as a quick reference guide to ensure that your note contains all of the essential elements.

	S: Subjective	
☐	1.	Use something significant the client says about his treatment or condition.
	O: Objective	
☐	1.	Begin this section with:
☐		○ Indication of active client engagement/participation
☐		○ Length of session
☐		○ Setting
☐		○ Purpose of session
☐	2.	Report your observations succinctly and accurately, either chronologically or using categories.
☐	3.	Remember to do the following:
☐		○ De-emphasize the treatment media
☐		○ Specify what part of the task required assistance
☐		○ Specify the exact type and amount of assistance needed
☐		○ Use professional language and standard abbreviations
☐		○ Show skilled OT happening
☐		○ Leave yourself out
☐		○ Focus on the client's response
☐		○ Avoid being judgmental
	A: Assessment	
☐	1.	Look at the data in your "S" and "O" sentence by sentence, asking yourself what problems, progress, and rehab potential you see.
☐	2.	Ask yourself, "So what? Why is this important in the client's life?" For each underlying factor not within functional limits, identify the impact it will have on an area of occupation.
☐	3.	End the "A" with *"Client would benefit from..."*
☐		○ Justify continued skilled OT
☐		○ Set up the plan
☐	4.	Be sure the time lines and activities you are putting in your plan match the skilled OT you indicate your client needs.
	P: Plan	
☐	1.	Specify the frequency and duration of OT treatment.
☐	2.	Tell what you will be working on during that time to address the client's needs.
☐	3.	Relate to a performance skill/area of occupation and client's OT goals.
☐	4.	Indicate any other pertinent follow-up needed for the client's present situation.
	Remember to:	
☐		Include the client's identifying information, delineate OT department and type of note.
☐		Correct errors properly, do not erase or use correction fluid, and do not leave blank spaces.
☐		Make certain engagement in occupation is integral to the note.
☐		Sign and date your note.

© SLACK Incorporated, 2013.

Morreale, M. J., & Borcherding, S. (2013). *The OTA's guide to documentation: Writing SOAP notes (3rd ed.).* Thorofare, NJ: SLACK Incorporated.

S: Subjective
- [ ] Use something **significant** the client says about his **treatment** or **condition**.
- [ ] If there is nothing significant, ask yourself whether you are using your interview skills to elicit the proper information about how the client sees things.

O: Objective
- [ ] Begin this section with length of session, where the client was seen, and for what purpose. Make sure you indicate active client participation. For example,
    Client participated in 30-minute OT session in hospital room for instruction in compensatory dressing techniques.
- [ ] Summarize what you see, either chronologically or using categories.
- [ ] Focus on performance skills and de-emphasize the treatment media. For example,
    Client worked on three-point pinch using pegs.
- [ ] Relate preparatory activities and physical agent modalities to occupational performance.
    Client worked on three-point pinch using pegs in order to manage buttons on clothing.
- [ ] Specify the **part** of the task needing assistance and the exact **type** and **amount** of assistance provided.
    Client required five verbal cues for correct hand placement during w/c ↔ toilet transfers.
- [ ] Indicate that the client **needed** assistance rather than labeling the client as an assist level.
    "Client required min assist..." rather than *"Client is min assist..."*
- [ ] Use standardized terminology to grade and describe treatment interventions and client performance.
- [ ] Show skilled OT happening—make it clear that you were not just a passive observer. For example, do not just list all of the assist levels and think that is enough.
- [ ] Write from the client's point of view, leaving yourself out.
    "Client was repositioned in w/c..." rather than *"COTA repositioned client in w/c..."*
- [ ] Focus on the client's response rather than on what you did.
    Client able to don socks using sock aid after demonstration.
- [ ] Avoid judging the client. For example,
    Say client *"...didn't complete the activity."* Don't add *"...because he was stubborn."*

A: Assessment
- [ ] Look at the data in your "S" and "O" sentence by sentence, identifying problems, progress, and rehab potential. Ask yourself what each statement means for the client's occupational performance. Consider the following formula:

Underlying Limiting Factor	Functional Impact	Ability to Engage in Occupation

  For example, if in your "O" you noted that client falls to the left when sitting unsupported, what do you think this means he will be unable to do for himself? For example,
    Client unable to sit EOB unsupported to dress.
- [ ] Make sure you have not introduced any new information.
- [ ] End the "A" with *"Client would benefit from..."*
- [ ] Justify continued skilled OT.
    Client would benefit from skilled instruction in use of adaptive devices and compensatory techniques for performing IADL tasks one-handed.
- [ ] Set up the plan and match time lines in your plan to the skilled OT you document that your client needs. For example, if you justify skilled OT by saying only, *"Client would benefit from skilled instruction in energy conservation techniques,"* then do not say that you plan to treat client twice a day for 2 weeks. Skilled instruction in energy conservation should take only one session or, at most, two sessions.

P: Plan
- [ ] Specify the frequency, duration of treatment, and specific OT interventions that will be implemented.
- [ ] Identify the performance skills and the areas of occupation that will be addressed during that time.
    Continue OT 1 hour daily for 2 weeks for upper body strengthening and instruction in adaptive devices needed for safe and Ⓘ transfers to bed, toilet, and tub.

© SLACK Incorporated, 2013.
Morreale, M. J., & Borcherding, S. (2013). *The OTA's guide to documentation: Writing SOAP notes (3rd ed.).* Thorofare, NJ: SLACK Incorporated.